I dedicate this book to my Uncle Sean.

The events in this book occurred between 2011-2014 all names and places have been anonymised for confidentiality.

Contents

Chapter 1: Nurse in London

Chapter 2: the weekend shift

Chapter 3: terror awaits

Chapter 4: nightmare lock-in

Chapter 5: Community nursing

Chapter 6: Jubilee Celebration

Chapter 7: Theatre

Chapter 8: Summer working have me a blast

Chapter 9: Final year: The cardiac ward

Chapter 10: The lift of terror

Chapter 11: Accident and emergency

Chapter 12: Casualty

Chapter 13: writer's life for me

Chapter 14 Top tips for student nurses

Prologue

They say that there are moments in our lives when an event occurs which shapes our destiny. When I was twelve years old and I went on a trip to Malvern, with my friend Jack, I discovered that I was meant to help people, I was destined for a career in a hospital setting.

It was the hottest August Sunday morning, and we rode our bikes around the hills. Jack was my closest friend, since I was four years old, and we enjoyed being around each other we enjoyed the same music, the same shows, and the same films.

On this morning, we were racing each other around the edges of the cliff, and suddenly Jack lost control of his bike and he jumped off and the bike went over the cliff. Jack held onto the edge of the cliff. I ran toward him and reached out my hands towards him. It was at that point I realized that if I let go, he would die.

"Please don't let go, Mark, I can't' die!" He shouted.

I could see the desperation in Jack, his face was sweating, and he managed to bring himself up from the edge. Jack's leg was cut deeply, and blood was oozing from the open wound. I quickly reached for the first aid box, and cleaned the wound with the antiseptic wipes, and wrapped the bandage around his leg compressing it. The ambulance team arrived ten minutes later and explained that my urgent assistance had been vital to saving Jack. A year later, Jack and his family died in a tragic plane crash. I was so thankful that I gave him an extra year, and I never had a good friend like Jack again. Jack had a huge influence on my decision to become a nurse.

Chapter 1: Nurse in London.

I arrived in central London in September, ready to commence my course. I left my suitcase in my new flat, whilst my four housemates were at work. It was a beautiful flat in canary wharf, with a beautiful view of the city. Inside the flat was a beautiful swirl pool, a games room, a balcony, and a luxurious dining room with a revolving sofa.

I spent my first-day sightseeing in London, I was finally feeling happy after surviving being attacked in my home city, I was feeling confident and safe again. I bought ice cream from the stand, I went onto the London eye and marvelled at how beautiful London looked, through the rays of the bright sun. I went to Madam Tussauds and enjoyed looking at the wax works.

"Wow he looks so realistic you almost think he is real," I smiled at a couple, as I looked at the elderly man standing like a statue. As the man moved forward, I jumped in shock, I thought he was a mannequin.

I then went to Bella Italia and I was very concerned when I had to wait an hour for my food. I was shocked when I arrived back at the flat and I found multi-coloured flowers and banners hanging on the ceiling.

"Welcome to the family," the flatmates shouted in unison. Mike was twenty-two, a music artist, and made a living from singing in pubs and singing at weddings. Mike was a wild character, often playing loud music and having wild parties. Martha was twenty-two and an actress, tanned, six-foot-tall with wild curly hair. Martha was very eccentric and would often wear wild outfits. Laura was twenty-four, a medical student, and was always locked away in her room, studying and appeared tearful most of the time. John was the oldest of the bunch at twenty-six, a lawyer who worked long hours, and like Mike, he too would hold large parties.

I started University in London the following day. The university I studied at was filled with students of a range of different ages. I sat next to Patti, in the lecture theatre, at the back. "Hi, I'm Mark, nice to meet you, I've just graduated from university."

"Hi, I am Patti, I have worked in healthcare all my life, and have just completed my health and social course."

I watched as Patti tucked into her boiling hot beef jerky and mash, the steam evaporated from the mash. I then sat through the lecture which was about the history of nursing. By the end of the lecture, Patti was fast asleep with her head tilted back snoring.

Four weeks later, I arrived at the Greet hospital for my first placement on a urology ward. I remember standing in the ward, I was petrified as I stood in my white student uniform, holding onto my notebook and pen in my hand. The ward was so busy, I could hear buzzers ringing, and patients shouting for help. The night nurses were rushing around, finishing their notes and completing their final duties. I then walked into the staff room for the handover. The ward manager stood up shaking my hand and giving me a beaming smile.

"Wonderful to meet you Mark, welcome to urology!" she smiled. I then observed Laurel and Hardy the healthcare assistants grunting in unison. The American nurse Ben and his colleague Cindy both smiled and shook my hand.

I then met my mentor Whitney a nurse, the same age as me, she was five months pregnant and had wild curly blonde hair, she appeared warm and friendly. I became confused during the handover, hearing words of salt and cabbage relating these to food, not knowing the correct medical abbreviations.

After the handover, I joined my mentor in the ward to meet my patients for the day. I was so terrified. I could feel my lips trembling, and I began to feel faint. "I'm ok," I repeated continuously to everyone who walked past.

I walked into my bay of male patients and looked on in awe at the patients. I was brand new, everything was new, and I had never looked after a sick person before. I looked after John a man living with prostate cancer and recovering from sepsis, Mat was admitted due to his dementia condition worsening and the care home struggling to support him. Then in the adjacent beds was Mick who was receiving chemotherapy treatment for lung cancer, David was admitted with a change in his diabetic condition, and Michael was awaiting to go home following his stay with pancreatitis.

I felt like a child on my first day at school, and Whitney decided I should get involved straight away. Whitney helped me to wash John whilst the healthcare assistant Debbie washed the other patients. We closed the hospital curtain and began to assist John with the wash. John required full assistance with washing, being turned in the bed, and required assistance with sitting up. John was at the end stage of his condition. I observed John's war medals attached to his bedside table, it was so sad to see him fighting his battle knowing how brave he was as a soldier. Throughout the day he would discuss stories from his time in battle.

After washing John, Whitney advised me to assist Mat with a wash whilst she attended the doctor's ward round. I had never interacted with a person living with dementia, I was nervous and worried. Mat sat in his chair in his chequered pyjamas next to the warm bowl of water.

"Who are you what are you doing here?" he shouted.

"I'm Mark, I'm a student nurse, I'm here to look after you," I began.

"I want to go home I don't like it here,"

"Well, you have to stay here Mat until you get better," I added.

Then as I turned around, I could see Mat's face was now boiling red, he held on tightly onto the bowl of warm water, I ducked as I threw the water over an unsuspecting Whitney.

As I walked out of the bay, I noticed the other patients had been washed, apart from David the 21-year-old diabetic patient who had the sheets wrapped around his head.

I then walked past Michael who grew impatient waiting for his tablets and discharge letter.

"Oi, you, I've been waiting almost two days for my tablets can you go and chase them up?"

"Yes, I will immediately I began." I walked over to the nurse's station to chase up information about the tablets. I looked around and felt overwhelmed by the busy atmosphere on the ward. The newly qualified nurse was stressed walking around with her giant medication trolley, desperate to complete the medication round on time, whilst a wet Whitney and ward manager Kate were walking with the consultant, carefully updating him on information about the patients' conditions.

Whitney had advised me to answer the buzzers of the patient. As a first-year student, I was able to enjoy talking to patients without completing the full responsibility. I walked over to John to help assist him with drinking his orange juice. John told me about how nervous he was at night kneeling in the trench on the outlook for the opposing army. John explained that during one attack as he ran to the oak tree, a young soldier jumped in front of John and another soldier, saving their lives whilst losing his own, it was his first night in the army, he was only seventeen years old, his life was just beginning.

I then answered the buzzer, it was Mick, Mick was exhausted following his chemotherapy treatment. I had to assist Mick with going to the toilet, I struggled as I helped to assist him out of the bed, and he stood with his walking stick. I suddenly had to check for hazards, whilst Matt repeatedly called me a bastard as I walked past. After I assisted Mick to the bathroom Whitney called me into the staffroom for our ward break. The ward manager Kate was an innovative manager who encouraged breaks for staff and supported their wellbeing. In the staffroom, Kate had prepared a dozen slices of toasts and several glasses of juice. I sat and gathered over ten pieces of toast and filled my glass with orange juice filled to the brim. The nurses laughed at me as I looked like a starving orphan.

"Glad to see you are settling in well," Katie smiled. The staff then sat around, giving updates on their patients in a relaxed and calm setting. I watched as Laurel and Hardy began to eat half of the sandwiches. It was great to be on such a supportive ward.

After I finished the ward meeting, I walked past the female bay and the women began to clap, and suddenly one of the women threw a pair of knickers at me which landed on my head, my face turned bright red with embarrassment.

It was then that Whitney ordered me to complete the observations on the patients. Every task I completed felt nerve-wracking, I was so nervous about making mistakes, I was looking for perfection knowing that I only had two weeks to complete. It was nerve-wracking being on the ward completing clinical tasks on the patients, after completing them on the mannequins.

I stood next to an already agitated Michael, as he now had waited more than twenty-four hours for his tablets. As I placed the blood pressure cuff on his arm I waited as it began to compress and to shock, it began to expand and attached from his arm. "Just go away," he groaned.

Whilst I completed Mick's observations, I became nervous as his five family members sat in their chairs all watching me, I felt under pressure and judged. I was pleased that the patients' observations were all stable a score of four or more in the observations would be a cause of concern.

I sat with Mat trying to support him trying to get to know what it is like to support someone living with dementia. Mat was sitting, colouring in the adult colouring book left by the ward.

"what are you colouring in?"

"None of your business!" John shouted.

"would you like me to get you a cup of tea?" I asked.

"Can I ask what you are doing here? You're walking around disturbing me I have all this work to do, and I've not got time to look after degenerates such as you," he warned. As I looked at the colouring book, I noticed that Mat had written numbers all over the booklet. Mat used to be an accountant and he believed that he was back at work.

Mat then explained that he needed the toilet and I helped him walk to the toilet. As I assisted him to the toilet, I wrapped the blue curtain around him. "I am just out here if you need me," I promised.

After Mat finished, he suddenly went quiet before storming through the curtain and grabbing me, throwing me against the wall, he slapped me across the face. "What is wrong with you? You will not leave me alone, keep away from me!" He roared.

"Help!" I shouted. Suddenly Laurel and Hardy came in to save the day, standing at either side of the mat calmly walking him back to his bed.

I felt I was drowning there was so much I needed to learn so much I had yet to experience.

I spent an hour with Whitney about the routines and tasks of the nurses on the ward. There were so many tasks including medication rounds, lunch rounds, and writing in notes, combined with the shortages in staff it made working on the ward very difficult.

That afternoon, I continued to support John who was having a bad day, he explained that he felt increasingly weak, he showed pictures from his photo album documenting his amazing life. From starting as a young soldier, to climbing up the ranks as general, to leave the army and training as a dentist, running his practice for over thirty years. It was clear to see the privilege nurses had in finding out about people's lives, and being part of their private moments. It was a privileged position.

I was exhausted by the end of the shift, I could feel my face burning red, Whitney sat me down by the nurse's station and took my temperature it was now over 40 degrees. Before the shift finished, we walked over to say goodbye to the patients, and I observed that John was in a deep sleep and when we looked closer, we realized he passed away. I felt a tear running down my eye. It was such an exhausting day; it opened my eyes to life working in healthcare. It was such a busy shift, I watched the nurses rushing around to complete deadlines, the healthcare assistants working desperately hard to make sure all patients were washed and that all their needs were met.

I returned to the flat that afternoon, I found it difficult adjusting to living with the housemates we were all so different. Martha had cooked us all a beautiful spaghetti bolognaise meal. Laura sat reading her medical book whilst John and Mike sat talking about football.

As we sat down for a meal Martha burst into tears crying as she was unsuccessful in an audition for a feature-length film, she had struggled after a month of auditions. I soon found that nursing was like a vocation, taking a strong commitment of twelve-hour shifts, sometimes working whilst skipping lunch.

Chapter 2: The weekend shift

At the start of each shift, I would feel nervous and apprehensive, each day on shift I felt like I was under a microscope being judged in everything I did. The first placement was based on understanding the basic needs of nursing, participating in personal care, completing clinical observations, and practicing my communication skills.

Whitney had assured me that the weekend shift was slower in pace, I was to find out that Whitney was desperately wrong.

I turned up the ward and it was so busy, the buzzers were constantly ringing, the night nurses were rushing around, desperately trying to finish their tasks for the night. I was less than relieved to see Laurel and Hardy working on the ward as they were so bossy and angry.

I was put into A bay which was known as 'the male bay,' the ward manager preferred for male students to look after male patients, which at the time felt like segregation from the female patients.

I walked with Whitney into the bay, and we met our five patients. The first patient was John a 90-year-old man with Dementia. John was admitted following worsening behaviour in the nursing home, and he sat with his bell from home.

The second patient was Chris, a 45-year-old man, admitted following worsening in his diabetes condition. Chris felt that his job as a Deputy Headteacher and the breakdown of his marriage contributed to a deterioration in his condition.

Thomas was a forty-year-old man, admitted from prison with pancreatitis. Thomas was very racist and projected racism towards staff.

Sean was admitted with chest pain and lived with autism; Sean was accompanied by his Mum who would provide him with emotional support. The fifth patient was eighty-nine-year-old John, admitted after a fall at home. John had a dressing across his head that he would frequently try and remove.

I watched each morning as Whitney intricately prepared her medication trolley preparing for the shift. As a student nurse, Whitney gave me a range of opportunities to administrate medications, through injection, and inhalers. I admired Whitney as she would spend time making sure that all the patients took their medication. Chris had begun to sing 'I will always love you,' something Whitney would experience frequently whilst giving her name to patients.

I spent ten minutes trying to encourage John to have his tablets, as John's dementia was advanced, he required verbal prompts to encourage him to take the medication.

I helped the patients set up for their morning wash with the help of Laurel and Hardy. Whitney had encouraged me to assist John with his wash, she wanted me to gain experience in supporting the patient with dementia.

"Hi John, is it ok if I help you with your wash?

"Yes Mr. Baldwin, you can help me, but this is not how we do it usually."

"No John I am not Mr. Baldwin; I am Mark the nurse."

"No, your Mr. Baldwin," he stated.

John believed that he was still in boarding school and believed that I was his previous headteacher. I had not yet gained the communication skills to effectively communicate with patients living with dementia. I assisted John by passing him the washcloth, and verbally instructed him to wash his face. Then when it came to assisting John with his shave disaster struck.

"What the hell are you doing?" he shouted. John pushed me away before emptying the bowl of water on his floor.

"I'm your nurse!" I panicked. Laurel and Hardy zoomed in, giving me a disconcerting look, before taking over the situation.

I then observed an angry Thomas sitting in his armchair handcuffed to the bed rails. "What are you looking at? You are fucking bastard!" He whined. I watched as the pharmacist began to complete notes at the end of his bed. "I wish people like you would go back to your home country, tell me did your Father set up an arranged marriage for you?" He barked. I watched as the pharmacist kept her cool, trying to ignore any retaliation to the racist insults. I quickly learned that in working in the NHS we had to accept all patients and accept discriminatory remarks from patients.

"Mark, I'm just going on a training course in the education centre for two hours, Sister Anne will be observing you," she smiled. I almost felt like I was attached to Whitney, I felt nervous if I was ever on my own. Whitney had instructed me to complete the clinical observations and update the care plans under the supervision of Sister Anne.

I carried the heavy observation machine ready to complete the observations. As I stepped towards John, I could see him holding his walking stick across his chest, "Come near me and it will be the last breath you take," he warned. I attempted to take the observations of Thomas, but he turned to me and frowned, "Just don't try it!" he barked.

"I will take his observations you take the observations of the other patients," Sister Anne smiled.

I walked over to Chris and watched as he sat in the chair looking distressed. I observed Chris looking at a picture of his ex-partner and his twin boys. As I took his observations, I discovered they were all in the normal ranges.

"that is a nice picture of your family," I smiled.

"Thanks' Mark, I had it all the perfect family my dream job and I lost it all because of one mistake!" he sighed.

"Maybe it is good for you now to take a step back, take some time out," I offered. As a nurse, I felt privileged to be able to support patients through their personal lives.

Sean's mother had to verbally prompt him to lift his arm and I could see that he did not feel comfortable with eye contact. As I took the observations, I could see that Sean was physically frightened holding onto his pillow. I soon realized that nothing could prepare me for my student nurse role, in looking after patients with a wide range of diverse conditions.

I then nervously walked over to John who sat with his head dressing in his hand. John had been living in his house on his own for thirty years, following the death of his wife. John's neighbour had reported concerns to social services a John was often found swearing and shouting at neighbours from his bedroom window. When John's house was investigated his house contained hundreds of rats scurrying around.

John's neighbour had helped him each week with his shopping effectively being the key person to keep him alive.

I had taken John's observation and his observations were in the normal parameter. Sister Anne had prepared the dressing, and I watched as he intricately placed the dressing on John's head.

Minutes later, I could hear John charging behind me with his Zimmer frame, as I turned around, I could see him standing with his dressing.

"Excuse me can you help me I found this?" he alerted, holding up his dressing.

I felt secure when Whitney returned to the ward, I almost felt like she was my safety blanket and was always there to assist me. I walked around my patients and began to check their end of bed notes, it was moments before lunch and the patients were relaxed and settled after a busy morning.

Then I walked over to Chris, and observed that he was sweating and began to slur his speech, he appeared confused and disorientated. I soon realized that Chris was having a hypoglycaemic attack. I ran to the nurse's station, for the diabetic emergency box, which contained glucagon and biscuits to help raise a person's blood sugar. I ran towards Chris with the box.

"well done Mark you were able to spot the emergency straight away." Sister Anne smiled.

As I put on my gloves, I opened the diabetic box and opened the gel and carefully applied it to Chris's gums, and passed him a small cup of orange juice. I slowly watched, as Chris regained consciousness, and his alertness improved.

"Thank you," Chris muttered. I could feel my heart pound against my chest, I was terrified of having to take the lead in an emergency.

Lunch was a very important time on the ward, we had to always ensure that patients were sitting upright and comfortable in their chairs.

I enjoyed giving out the meals, as I was able to meet the patients in other bays. I watched as Whitney sat in her chair at eye level helping to feed John his warm roast dinner meal. John gave Whitney a concerned look, "Who is that weird person? He says his name is Mark, is there anyone that can take him for mental examination?" he asked.

At lunch, I went to the cafeteria and sat next to two students on my course, Rakel, and Susan. Rakel had over twenty years' experience as a carer and had explained that her placement was 'like a walk in the park,' and 'too easy' for her. Susan felt she was struggling on the AMU ward as her mentor was a senior charge nurse and she felt constantly tested and out of her depth. It was clear to see that we all had different experiences as student nurses.

When I returned to the ward, I could see a stressed Whitney standing at the nurse station.

"Mark, I need your help, I need you to stay in the bay to look after John, he has had an angry episode earlier and requires one-to-one supervision, update the bed notes, and take the observations. I noticed that the curtains were wrapped around Thomas, he had an angry outburst on the ward and refused to speak to other staff members. Chris was exhausted from his previous emergency episode. Sean has discharged, and it now unusually quiet on the ward, a peace that I cherished. I had managed to update the skin charts, the fluid charts, and bed lists, I also managed to write in my reflective journal.

I tried desperately not to wake John up almost tiptoeing around the ward to avoid waking him. Then disaster struck, as I stood up, I knocked into the bedside table causing the water jug to crash onto the floor. John bolted up from the bed in shock.

"what's going on? Who are you? Where is my mother?"

"I am the student nurse here to help you today," I replied.

"Help!" John roared at the top of his lungs. Whitney zoomed into the ward and helped him to remain calm.

During the eight-week placement, Whitney and the staff fully supported me in helping to orientate me to the ward, I was able to learn the basics of nursing care, and shadowing and capturing ideas from other nurses helped to inform my own practice.

At the end of the placement, I joined my housemates on a day trip to Alton towers, it was the first time we were all together as a group. John took us in his jeep, and we all looked forward to the fun-filled day. Martha was on the phone throughout the journey talking to her agent, looking for new opportunities in her acting roles. Laura was sitting at the back quietly reading her book, even on her day off she struggled to unwind and switch off from work, Mike was trying to coax everyone into a singing foreigner, 'I want to know what love is,' whilst I sat quietly listening to my podcasts.

We arrived at the theme park at 10 am, and the first ride we went on was the smiler ride. As we on the ride I could hear Martha screaming at the top of her lungs. I felt so dizzy and sick as my head banged from side to side. As the ride finished, I struggled to walk off with Laura who stumbled and held onto my arm. As we exited the ride, we witnessed the smiler spinning sign spinning on the wall, it made me feel so weak and dizzy, so I knelt beside the bench in desperation. Mike and John felt it would be funny to carry me by my legs and my arms around the park. After half an hour, I drank a refreshing glass of water which helped to alleviate my fears.

The next ride we went on was the log flume, as a group, and disaster struck when Martha lost her diamond ring, she began to scream hysterically, she splashed her hand desperately in the water, but she struggled to find it.

After, we went on the Halloween maze. I was terrified as we walked through the maze it was a dark pitch-black tunnel with fading white lights. I could hear eerie music playing in the background and the sound of a wolf howling. As I walked through the maze, I could feel breathing on my neck. Suddenly I felt two zombie arms reaching out at me and I could see the green furry hands reaching out grabbing me. As we reached the end of the tunnel, we reached a lift. As we entered the lift, we could hear a loud shrill scream, then a white light turned on showing a beheaded zombie holding a head in his hand.

After the ride, Mike decided to buy us all an ice cream sundae and we enjoyed basking in the sun. We then all glided along with the ice rink, it was the perfect end to a break away from my life on the ward. it is so important as a student nurse to take breaks away, and enjoy your free time.

Chapter 3: Terror awaits

I started my second placement in an acute medical ward. Being a student nurse can be very difficult and adapting to a new ward can bring challenges. My new mentor was Kate, a sixty-year-old nurse, with over forty years in the NHS. Kate was always busy, and was the student coordinator, and expected students to adapt very quickly with little support. Gill the ward manager trained with Kate and was very hands-on, and would often work alongside nurses to help them achieve their targets. Suki the nurse associate was very sarcastic and despised working with 'student's, which made it difficult to work alongside her.

My first shift was manic, and I realized I was caring for patients who required close observation and monitoring. As we completed the medication round, Kate explained her expectations for me as a student.

"Well now that you are in a second placement you need to move beyond the basics of nursing, I want you now to focus on assessing deteriorating patients and acting on patient observations," She smiled. Kate was very busy as a nurse, and very systematic in her approach in supporting students, she would set clear targets.

The first patient I was supporting was John, who was admitted with shortness of breath and was a previous army veteran. John required close observation due to his confusion and his habit of removing his mask.

The second patient was Mike a one-hundred-year-old man, living with dementia admitted with recurrent UTIs. Mike was well known for his aggressive behaviour and would often throw items at patients.

Thomas was 90 years old and was recovering after being admitted following a stroke. Thomas required full assistance with turning and moving in the bed.

Martin was fifty-four, and required one-to-one supervision admitting following a worsening in his brain cancer illness which had now reached grade 4.

Sean was admitted following an infection in his legs which led to sepsis. Sean was alerted to social services after setting his kitchen on fire. Sean was very unkempt, and his clothes were dirty, and he refused to take part in any personal care.

The final patient was Sara, a thirty-five-year-old woman, admitted with a sudden change in her diabetes condition.

After the medication round, Kate had brought several washing bowls ready for me to wash the patients, I had a strong feeling the shift would be difficult.

I walked over to mike, "Hi Mike I am Mark a student nurse, Can I assist you with a wash this morning?"

"Come near me again and I will break your fingers!" he groaned. I was happy when Kate offered to wash Mike.

I then assisted John with his wash, it was so nice to see the old photo of him standing with his wife on their wedding day in his army outfit. It was great to see the life of patients and to get to know their backgrounds. John was very breathless throughout his wash constantly pulling his mask off his face, being too weak to fully move, I felt it was best for him to stay in bed for the morning.

"John please keep your mask on it is helping you to breathe," I warned. I alerted Kate as his breath became more laboured.

I then went to assist Martin with a wash, Martin was a retired headteacher but left shortly after his cancer diagnosis. As I assisted him with a wash, I noticed how confused he was. Martin began to slur his speech and appeared muddled in his thoughts.

"where am I, why am I here? When can I go home?" Then by the end of the wash and dressing assessment, Martin was more coherent in his speaking and was able to speak about his role as a headteacher.

When I finished supporting Martin with his wash, I had walked out to find all the patients sitting in their chairs and all the beds looking smart. Suki the arrogant HCA called me into the sluice room.

"Hi Mark, I need to tell you I think you are too slow, and you are too shy, on this ward you will not survive on the ward unless you change. Ok?

"ok" I answered.

As I walked out into the bay, I could see the consultant Dr. Geoffrey talking to Sean asking him questions testing to see if he was confused.

"What year is it?"

"1825"

Where are you?"

"Fuck you, what are you asking questions for?

"Sir I do not appreciate that language I am the consultant. I understand you have been living in your house on your own for forty years, are you aware of the infestation of rats?"

"My goodness you are such a nosy bastard, my life is none of your business now keep away!" he yelled.

Doctor Geoffrey had organized for the mental health team to come to the ward to assess him as he needed help.

Doctor Geoffrey then observed Martin sleeping, and he stood with the multi-disciplinary team talking about his latest test results. Doctor Geoffrey stated that Martin's cancer had progressed further and had spread to his vital organs, giving him a prognosis of only one month.

After the round, Kate asked me to complete the observations of the patients. As I walked up to Mike, he gave me a startled look and grabbed the fruit from his bowl. First, he threw the apple narrowly missing me, then the pair, and thirdly the oranges. I managed to duck. As Suki walked in, Mike threw the jig of water at her, soaking her completely.

"Oh, Mike how could you this? This will stain!" she roared. I was happy that Suki had got her just deserts.

I then took Sean's observations, I struggled to stand by him with the smell of faeces from his dirty clothes.

"How do you feel? It seems like you had a difficult conversation with Dr. Geoffrey?"

"Well Mark, the doctors simply do not understand my wife and daughter died in an accident forty years ago. It is not easy living on your own, but I am making the best of it. I just hope they do not take my home from me," he urged. It was clear to see that Sean had lived a very difficult life which led to him not preserving his self-care.

I then went to take Jack's observations, I could see already that his physical presentation showed that he was in distress. John's shoulders were moving rapidly up and down, his breaths were over 30 a minute, his heart rate was over 100 beats per minute. Jack shouted for help, and I pressed the emergency buzzer as he became unresponsive. Kate, Gill, and all the ward staff arrived at his bed.

Kate tried to see if Jack responded to touch and rested her ear on him to see if he was breathing, she ordered me to run for the crash trolley. I rushed to the corner of the ward grabbing the trolley, sweating with nerves. When I arrived back in the bay, I observed Kate completing the thirty chest compressions, and putting the oxygen mask onto his face administrating two breaths. I watched as Doctor Geoffrey completed the compression as the cardiac lead practitioner shouted orders. I watched as the ward manager, Gill, placed the defibrillator on him administrating the shock. It was of no use. Jack died minutes later, as a student, I felt immediate guilt. What did I do wrong? What could I do better?

I watched as the team slowly disappeared, and we had to prepare Jack and complete the 'last offices' a procedure, in which deceased patients are prepared for going to the morgue. I felt so emotional during the procedure, I felt I was fighting back the tears, here was Jack sitting in the chair only an hour later to now having passed away. I watched in shock as the ward manager Gail ordered us to clear the bed for an incoming patient, this was the NHS there was no time to mourn the loss of a patient you had to remain resilient. I was thankful for a ten-minute tea break which helped me to collet my thoughts.

I then walked into the side room to find Sally crying in the bed in her pink nightgown.

"What wrong?" I asked.

"I have just had a review by the doctor, and I have discovered that I am pregnant with twins. My partner has left me, I do not feel capable to look after a child.

"Is there anything I can do?" I asked.

"just go!" She warned.

As I walked out of the side room I was overwhelmed with the busy nature of the ward. The ward was filled with healthcare professionals. The physiotherapists were mobilizing patients, the occupational therapists were completing kitchen assessments, and the nurses were rushing around to complete notes assessments and discharges. Each shift as a student nurse was different from the next, and today it felt like a manic atmosphere.

Mrs. Rhodes wife of Martin had arrived to speak with the consultant Mr. Geoffrey and My mentor Kate to reveal the diagnosis. It was very difficult sitting in the cold blue clinical room. Mrs. Rhodes sat in her bright blue coat with her hair in rollers.

"I'm so sorry Mrs. Rhodes but cancer has now spread, and you may want to consider immediate hospice care."

I could see the look of devastation wash over Mrs. Rhodes her calm exterior dissolved, she broke down into a flood of tears.

"I had so much planned for us, I thought we would have time to have a summer together on the beach, we have been together since we were sixteen, I can't cope without him!" she cried. I watched as Kate reached out her hand to Mrs. Rhodes.

As I walked back into the bay, I could see Martin talking to his friend his ex-colleague Simon. I could see Martin smiling and nodding politely to Simon. Then as Simon left, I could see a glazed look edged on his face.

"Martin, what's Wong?"

"I am devastated I can not even remember who that man is I had to pretend that I knew what he was talking about."

I watched as Simon broke down in tears.

"I'm so scared," he gasped.

"We are here for you; your wife is in the relative room would you like to see her?" I smiled, reaching out my hand to Martin. I walked with Simon into the bathroom, and I had to guide him by his hands as he struggled to walk, the part of his brain which controlled movement was affected by the tumour. As Simon reached the relative's room, he cradled his distraught wife.

I reached the ward to complete the afternoon observations and looked on in laughter. From the window of the bay, I could see Mike throwing contents from Thomas's table at Suki, it seemed like justice prevailed.

Chapter 4: Nightmare lock-in

I was finally settling into life as a student nurse, I felt part of the team, I had my locker, the staff knew my name and I had completed many of my competencies. I was about to complete one of my first nightshifts. I had packed so much in my rucksack, toothpaste, and toothbrush, sandwiched, a bottled fizzy drink, and several packets of crisps. I needed to stay alert I had to get through the shift.

At the start of the shift, Whitney asked me to go to the linen cupboard after the night shift to collect a basket of linen. I walked into the room at the end of the corridor, and as I stepped in, I grabbed the trolley. The door was locked behind me, I was locked in.

This was my worst nightmare being tapped in a small room, I began to bang the doors shouting for help, "let me out I'm a student nurse I am trapped!" I shouted in desperation. My phone was in my jacket in the staffroom I started to panic. The room was right outside the accident and emergency waiting room area, I was locked in for two hours before the light turned off. I repeatedly started to bang the door whenever I heard footsteps going past. I wondered why no one answered, I was terrified with no idea that the wall was soundproofed. That night, I could hear the conversation as I walked past. I could hear a desperate husband waiting for the news of his wife who was undergoing an emergency caesarean operation. Each time a nurse or doctor walked out of the operating room he would shout out, "Any news? How is she?" Then a half an hour I could hear a nurse shout, "it's a girl!"

I then hear a young woman crying as she had taken a fall downstairs after tripping on a laptop in the night. "Help me I think I have broken my foot," she shouted coming through the doors, "You're going to be alright," her boyfriend urged. "Shut up it was your fault you left the laptop on the stairs!" she yelled.

I could then hear a woman crying talking to her mother right outside the room.

"We are going to get you the help you need now, this can't go on any longer, you sleep all day you never go out."

"I miss Dad so much life is so hard without him, everything changed when he died," she gasped.

"I miss your father too, but you have to try to move on with your life, your nineteen, you should be starting at work or going to university. We are not leaving here until you get help!" She warned.

I could hear a newborn parent's family waiting anxiously as she was admitted with a high temperature. I was exhausted, I felt like I had been trapped in the room forever, I collapsed into deep sleep.

The next morning, I was awoken by a nurse who entered the room letting out a terrified scream. "Security! There is an intruder in the cloakroom, please help," she yelled.

I came back to the ward at 7 am to a concerned Kate, "Where the hell have you been?"

"It was a nightmare I was locked in the cloakroom all night.

My second placement in the acute medical ward was full of challenges. Kate was a strict but fair mentor she imparted her knowledge and gave me plenty of clinical opportunities to learn nursing skills. In my second placement, I learned how to respond to a deteriorating patient, how to respond to cardiac emergencies, and the role of the wider multi-disciplinary team. I still however felt like a nurse baby. I had so much more left to learn.

That summer I decided to go to Northumberland on holiday, I needed a break after a stressful year. I stayed at my Grandparents' house which was right at the edge overlooking the beach. The scenic stone cottage overlooked the crystal sea and the bright sand. Inside the cabin was a beautiful grand white piano, the conservatory let to the balcony which wooden steps leading to the beach. The golden spiral staircase led to the beautiful king-size bed. At night I would listen to the choir of crickets and the sound of the crashing of the waves. I missed my Grandparents so much, I had so many positive memories of the time I spent at the beach, My Grandparents had taught me how to swim, we had jumped from the cliff edge into the beautiful sea.

During the day, I would sit on my sun lounger and see the same people on the beach. Mrs. Daisy would walk along the beach with her black Labradors wearing her red coat. Each day, Daisy would buy me ice cream. Then I spoke to Sean Malley, a local fisherman who would talk to me about football and film. I observed Karen and Sara the twins who lived a mile from the cottage playing tennis at the centre of the beach. The girls were the same age as me and I watched them grow up. Sara was competitive, and outgoing, whilst Karen was shy and far more reserved. The people in Northumberland appeared more outgoing and positive than the people in Birmingham.

I would spend hours sitting on the sun lounger writing in my journal allowing me to escape into another world.

That night, the one peaceful retreat I once knew was about to turn into a nightmare.

I was watching my favourite film Edward Scissorhands and sat on the revolving sofa eating my home-baked lasagne with pretzel cheese. It was the perfect relaxing night, as I looked out of the window, I could see the moon was full and bright, possibly a sign that something bad was about to happen.

As I walked up the spiral staircase, I could hear a faint cry in the distance. At first, I thought it was my imagination but slowly the screams and shouts for help grew louder and louder.

I knew that I needed to go and help the distressed person. As I arrived on the beach and I looked out into the distance hoping to see through the light of the moonlight, a faint image of a person crying for help. I decided to climb up the mountain top so I could have a better view. As I reached the top and I could visibly see someone splashing in the sea, "Help," she shouted. It was then that I called the ambulance, I took a jump back and I dived into the sea. As I crashed into the sea as I swam desperately in the sea, I found the person's hand and slowly pulled the person up, it was Karen, one of the twins I met at the beach.

"Please help me I do not want to die!" she stammered. I pulled Karen along the sea with all my strength as Karen became weaker and weaker.

I could hear her cry faintly, "I want to live," she gasped. As I helped Karen up to the edge, I realized she was unconscious. I immediately undertook CPR, but it was no use Karen died at the scene. I was taken into the ambulance in shock. Every time I felt I was relaxed or happy something would come along and disrupt my life.

Chapter 5: Community nursing

After an intense and eventful summer, I was happy to return to university it felt like I was returning to normality. My second year was more intense in content and we learned how to support patients in the community, pregnant mothers, and how to support patients with illnesses such as cancer and diabetes. Over twenty students had dropped out from the course after the intensity of the first-year placement, and it was common for a high percentage of students to drop out.

I was nervous as I arrived at the nursing reception desk to discover my placement allocation. I was allocated to working with a small virtual ward community team. The community virtual ward had one primary aim, to support patients on discharge and prevent readmission into hospitals.

The virtual nurse team was made up of nurses, doctors two physiotherapists, and a consultant.

My mentor was Louise a former beautician, who gave me a glazed confused expression.

"Hi, I'm Louise I'm your mentor, you're my first ever student," she smiled nervously, I could see that Louise had reluctantly accepted the role of mentor. I sat next to Debbie, a community matron with over thirty years of experience in the NHS. The healthcare assistant Sharon was training to be an assistant practitioner and was able to complete advanced clinical duties, such as taking blood and completing compression dressings. It was great to be so welcomed into the district nurse team, I was given a warm cup of tea, my desk, and my locker, a world away from being given a draw in the cabinet for all my belongings.

Louise collected her dressings folder and other nursing supplies and we walked to her car. Louise showed me the list of patients we were going to see. The patients had a range of conditions from diabetes, dementia, to terminal cancer.

As we reached the carpet, I looked on in awe at Louise's car a red Porsche. As I climbed in Louise zoomed out of the car park. Louise explained that she had worked as a beautician for over fifteen years before training as a nurse at thirty-five, she repeatedly told me that she was nervous about having a student. Before we arrived at the first house Louise drove to Tesco to buy a box of gloves.

"Right Mark I will only be ten minutes stay here don't touch anything," she warned. After five minutes of waiting, I pressed the button for the radio but of course, it was the wrong button. Suddenly the alarms went off in the car and it sounded like a police siren. Suddenly shoppers rushed out of the shop including the ward manager. Louise walked back to the car and gave me a concerned look; I had made such a bad impression on my first day!

The first house we visited was Donald an eighty-nine-year-old man, who was admitted to hospital after fainting at home, it was later discovered that he had developed diabetes type 2. We opened the door and Donald invited us into his Elvis-themed dining room. All over the walls were pictures of Elvis throughout his career, and on the walls were framed Elvis disks. Several Elvis cut-outs were placed around the room, it felt overwhelming.

"Wonderful to meet you, Donald, how are you coping with your new diabetic diet?" Louise asked.

"It's going ok, I have reduced my calorie intake and sugar consumption. Do you want to look into my fridge I can show you, my diet?"

We walked over to the fridge and looked on in terror. The fridge was filled with three chocolate homemade cakes, five bottles of coke, and a dozen cheese sandwiches.

"I stick to sandwiches instead of pizza for Lunch, then just one whole cake a day," he explained. As we moved back to the living room Louise took Donald's blood sugar reading which was very high. Louise issued a good diet guide that shows the number of carbohydrates and fats he could have.

"Donald, I must tell you I am concerned about your blood sugar reading, and your diet it puts you at significant risk," Louise explained.

I have found the diagnosis very hard to cope with, and I have just lost my job I'm struggling and because I'm on my own the food is my only comfort," he stammered as tears rolled down his eyes. Louise had offered Donald talking therapy to talk through his illness and to help him to terms with his condition. It was clear to see that Donald had struggled due to lifestyle factors in controlling his condition.

We then visited 95-year-old Samantha's grand mansion. Samantha was diagnosed with terminal lung cancer, and we arrived to offer her intravenous medication. The house was four stories high with a thirty-acre garden a swimming pool tennis court. Inside the house was a personal cinema room, a grand dance hall, and upstairs there were fifteen rooms. As we made our way into the house, we marvelled at the photos on the wall. Samantha was a famous makeup artist to the stars and the pictures on the wall included her standing with Madonna, Steven Spielberg, and Michael Jackson.

Samantha had contributed to the make up for over fifty film productions. Samantha had been married to Bill for seventy years, and he sadly passed away together they fostered over one hundred children together.

It was such a privilege working in the community and gaining an insight into the personal lives of patients. As we walked up to the spiral staircase, I marvelled at the beautiful paintings as we walked to the end of the corridor to Samantha's room. Samantha was laying in her beautiful king-size bed overlooking her beautiful scenic garden, lying next to her were her two corgis. I watched as Samantha administrated the end-of-life medications through the syringe driver.

"You have a wonderful house; it looks like you've had a wonderful career." I smiled.

"Well, it was wonderful getting the opportunities to work on amazing films like Jaws and Indiana Jones, I got to travel the world and meet famous people, I constantly felt like I was living a dream. I came over here with my parents from Germany we were immigrants and so poor." She explained.

Samantha played her classical music on her stereo in the corner of the room she had a stack of her favourite novels.

"It is so great to see you smiling Sam, you're an inspiration," Louise explained.

"Well, you have to keep positive, many of my friends and family have passed, and I'm just grateful for each day I have, each day I watch home videos from my time as a makeup artist, it is wonderful to have positive memories." She smiled.

It was great to see how positive Samantha was, her room was filled with flowers and gifts from her Grandchildren and friends showing their support. The medications administrated to Samantha gave her comfort in her final days.

We then travelled to see Ajar, an 80-year-old man, who had been admitted to hospital with severe panic attacks and anxiety following an attack at his local shopping centre. When we arrived at the house, we witnessed over ten cars on the driveway. We knocked on the door and Mr. Ajars wife arrived wearing a bright red dress and a part hat.

"Oh, Louise and Boy, wonderful to see you it is Ajar's birthday today, I know he will be simply thrilled to see you.

"Oh, we don't want to disturb you, we can come back another day," Louise explained.

"nonsense," Anne smiled, ushering us both into the house. I looked on in shock the house was filled with hundreds of guests dancing to bhangra music surrounded by balloons and confetti. It showed the unpredictable nature of community nursing. As we reached the conservatory, we observed Ajar cutting the cake in the room smiling at the guests. "Mr.

Ajar It is great to see you so happy, we came to review but we will come to see you another day," Louise explained. Mrs. Ajar nearly forced us to sit on the sofa and gave us a plateful of sandwiches and crisps and a soda drink. Louise had offered to put the candles on the cake, and everyone cheered as she walked out of the room. It truly showed how you could never predict what happens in the community settings.

We then carried onto the next house, a seventy-nine-year-old man called Gerald who was living with dementia, and his eighty-year-old wife Deborah was struggling to support him as the main carer.

As we drove along in the Porsche, Louise began to talk to her husband in the car putting him on speakerphone, I felt instantly uncomfortable as they spoke affectionately.

"I love you honey poos," Louise gushed,

"Love you too fatty," Mark replied.

We arrived at Gerald's thatched Edwardian cottage at 1 pm and we found a distraught Deborah standing outside, her whole body was trembling.

"Oh, Louise I am so glad you're here I am having a really difficult morning, I can't get Thomas up from the kitchen floor he is refusing!" she panicked. We rushed into the kitchen and found Gerald laying on the floor his expression was glazed, and he appeared confused.

"Hi, Gerald. We are from the virtual ward team we are here to help you can you stand up for us please?" Louise asked.

We watched as Deborah carried a standing frame and put it in front of Gerald, placing his hand on the frame, and putting her arm under his shoulders.

"C'mon Gerald stand up you can do this, he usually stands with the frame," Deborah explained. We could see that Deborah was physically struggling as the carer, and she showed how vulnerable she was.

"Deborah, we need to call the ambulance Gerald is in distress and we can't leave him on the floor," Louise stated.

"No, you can't call the ambulance they will take him away from me!" Deborah roared.

"No, you both need help. This is not safe, he can't just be left on the floor," Louise warned.

"He will get up eventually, sometimes he falls in the bathroom, but he gets up in his own time," she added.

The ambulance team came and used a hoist to help Gerald onto the hospital trolley. Gerald required an assessment of his care needs, and

Deborah broke down in tears as she guided him by the hands into the ambulance. It was interesting to see as a student the journey of people living with dementia, and just how tough life can be as a carer for someone living with dementia.

We then visited the next house, Barbara Wilson required honey dressings on her legs. When we stepped into the house, we could see thousands of OK magazines which filled up the living room. Barbara was a big fan of the magazine. The only interaction Barbara would have been with the district nurse team, the magazines were her only comfort. At first, Barbara consented for me to complete the dressing then halfway through the dressing she began to shout, "I don't want Mark to help me, I remember I don't really like students," she shouted out. This was the unpredictable nature of being a student.

I came home to the apartment that night and walked into a wild party hosted by Mike and John, Martha and Laura were away, and they were using their free time to hold lavish parties. I was exhausted and collapsed into my bed.

Working in the community setting was less intense than working on the ward. I felt the work-life balance was more sustainable, the hours were shorter, and staff appeared closer and more supportive. I felt that Samantha was very disconnected from her role as a mentor, some nurses are natural teachers, and it was clear to see that Samantha struggled in her role.

I was invited to take part in completing a night shift with 60-year-old experienced nurse Gill. Gill had worked as a community nurse for over forty years with the district nurse team. Gill was eccentric a chronic smoker, funny, and built a great rapport with all the patients she met.

I arrived at the district nurse's office at 7am and we drove in Gill's jeep. I felt like I was choking as she smoked throughout the journey.

"Do you enjoy working in the community do you miss working on the ward?" I asked.

"I love working in the community as I have a caseload of patients that I have known for years, I care about them, and sometimes I am the only contact for my patients. I love the variety of working in clinics supporting pregnant patients, children, and patients with a range of long-term illnesses and I get to provide patient education." She smiled.

It was clear to see that Gill had vast experience and so much to offer students. I was so nervous at her terrible driving skill, she would drive on the pavement and constantly beep her horn at anyone who drove past, I felt like a nervous wreck as we drove along the motorway.

The patient we went to was Daisy an eighty-five-year-old lady who required her insulin injection. Daisy lives with her 99-year-old husband David who was fast asleep in his armchair. When we walked into the house, we observed a tearful Daisy crying in her armchair, whilst her husband David was snoring next to her.

"Oh, it is wonderful to see you Gill it has been a tough week. I just feel that David is not interested in me he spends most of his time sleeping," she cried.

"Well Daisy he is 99, maybe he needs a lot of sleep," Gill explained, whilst embracing Daisy.

"I don't want him to leave me, I can't cope without him!" she shouted.

Gill administrated the insulin injection Daisy and Gill was soon able to calm her nerves. As we left the room David pinched Gill on her bottom with one eye open!

Various risks were working in the evening and night shifts. Gill explained that previously she had her car stolen from visiting a house and her phone snatched. As we walked out of the house, we had noticed a gang of teenagers hanging around at the street corner and we both felt nervous.

"I'm sure they put me on the evening shift as they don't mind bumping off the old lady!" she joked.

"How are you finding the course? Are you enjoying your time with us? You do appear nervous sometimes," She began.

"I'm nervous with the unknown, I was just getting used to the hectic environment with the wards then I'm sent to the community."

"You will get there but you must utilize all your placements as learning opportunities ask to be part of as many clinical duties as you can," Gill warned.

We then arrived at Bethany's house, a seventy-eight-year-old lady, who requested the flu vaccine. Gill asked me to administrate the injection and I was excited to finally be given the chance to be involved in clinical skills.

"Right, we should only be in here for ten minutes, Bethany has a habit of talking for long periods, so we have to be very direct. When we entered the house Bethany, and her husband Derek was very welcoming and asked us for a cup of tea to which we refused. I felt my fingers trembling as I held the injection in my hand.

"Oh, bless him he only looks twelve, he is so cute, oh bless he is going red!" she laughed. I injected Bethany with her injection and after she let out a scream. I was startled and both Bethany and Gill laughed at my nervousness. As we sat on the couch Derek walked out with two cups of tea and a tray of cake.

"You both can't leave without a cup of tea! He smiled.

"Oh, go on can't say no!" Gill smiled rolling her eyes. The plan to stay for ten minutes soon went out the window and Gill spoke about every topic from the weather to the plot of EastEnders. As I sat on the couch, I could feel the eyes of her pit bull terrier digging into mine as he sat staring at me, I remained still, and in desperation, I threw a piece of cake on the floor to divert his attention.

The final house of the night was Michael a 30-year-old man who lives with schizophrenia who was recently discharged from hospital after making a suicide attempt. We were visiting Michael to see how well he was adjusting to life at home. When Michael opened the door to his flat, he was dressed in a green florescent tracksuit, his house was filthy with pizza boxes, sweet wrappers, and laundry scattered across the floor.

"Oh, Michael you need to get help with your house we can assist you with his." She smiled.

"How have you been?" Gill asked.

"Before we talk there is something I want to show you both in the broom cupboard. We both stepped into the cupboard and as soon as we entered Michael closed the door and locked us in.

"Ha Ha now you can't get out," he murmured.

"Oh, fucking hell!" Gill muttered.

"Please tell me we are not locked in?" I gasped.

"We can get round this," Gill began.

"This is a really fun game, but I have snakes and ladders in the car we can play that?" Gill offered.

"You judged me as soon as I entered the house, you said it was messy everyone is judging me all the time," he sobbed.

I witnessed Gill texting the emergency mental health crisis team to come to the house. Ten minutes later, the team arrived and completed an assessment. It was a nerve-wracking experience, but it showed the risks and unpredictable nature of working in the community. I passed my community nursing placement, although I felt I gained more experience in my communication skills than my clinical skills. I received my next allocation, and discovered I was going to be sent to a theatre department next.

Chapter 6: Jubilee celebration

Before I commenced my theatre placement, I was happy to participate in the jubilee celebrations, and I invited my flatmates to Birmingham to participate in the celebration. I was so excited when I woke up in the morning, and found a table covering the width of the road on the street. On the table was an English flag tablecloth. On the lampposts, the British flags hung on each one. My neighbours slowly came out and brought out a range of food, sandwiches, pizza, and chocolates. The street was running an amazing cake celebration. One cake was made in the shape of the Queen's crown, whilst another cake was a five-tier fruit cake, and at the top were edible caricatures of the royal family.

I was shocked when I witnessed John and Mike dressed in sumo wrestler outfits wearing the masks of Prince Charles. Martha helped me in the kitchen in the morning to help make our last-minute jubilee cake. In her typical fashion, Laura was already sitting at the table reading her Agatha Christie novel. It was the most beautiful sunny day; it was great to have a break from the intense nature of the nursing course.

Mum and Dad had given us all union jack suits to wear and my Dad oversaw the music and brought his cd with a range of music from the 70's to the present. After an hour, we took the cake out of the oven and Martha spent time putting the icing on the cake, and we displayed it on the kitchen table. Everything was going well, too well……

I returned to the kitchen and the cake was destroyed and my dog Rex was covered in cake licking her lips and Martha was traumatized.

When we walked onto the street, we were mesmerized by the happy atmosphere hearing everyone laughing. As we sat down everyone completed the Mexican wave led by Mike and John. Then Mike led everyone into a singsong, and we sang 'sweet Caroline,' together.

It was the perfect day; the food was delicious, and I could feel a strong community feel. It was amazing to sing the bohemian rhapsody together in unison. Then Mike stood on the table and shouted, "C'mon everyone it's time to do the conga!" he yelled. John played the conga song by black lace and like that Mike started off the conga line I linked myself to Martha and joined the conga line we danced around the table, singing together, it was a magical moment.

It was a wonderful afternoon, and we enjoyed consuming our cake together. I was having the perfect break from my studies and thought that everything was going well until an emergency occurred.

I could hear screaming at the end of the table, it was Judy and Alex the young couple who lived on the corner of the street. I could see that Judy's eleven-year-old daughter Hayley was collapsed on the floor.

"She's been stung by a bee can anyone help?"

I looked at Hayley's face her lips were swollen, she was struggling to breathe, "Call the ambulance she has had an anaphylactic shock," I warned. Judy ran back into her house and grabbed the anaphylactic treatment box.

"I have the injection, but I can't remember how to use it!" Judy panicked.

I grabbed the EpiPen and administrated the injection which contained adrenaline, which helped reverse the adverse effects of the sting.

The ambulance team arrived and assessed Hayley at the roadside and applied oxygen.

"Well done Mark you saved Hayley's life you acted fast and that's just what you needed to do." She murmured.

Whilst I enjoyed the day with my family, I felt like I could not escape my life as a student nurse.

Chapter 7: Theatre

I commenced the theatre placement, on the following Monday, at a small private hospital near the countryside. The private hospital was made of a close-knit team of forty staff including nurses, Operating department practitioners, and surgeons. On appearance, it felt like a happy environment, but I had no idea that I had just walked into hell. I had two mentors Sally, a sixty-year-old Sister, and Dawn the nurse who would make my life a living hell as a student nurse. Dawn had red hair and wore a green belt. Dawn had openly admitted to me and other staff that she disliked being a mentor, and felt that students were not suited to being in the theatre department.

On the first few days in the theatre, I was asked to observe surgery and observe the pathway of patients in the department. I followed a patient having a new knee replacement. It was cold and uncomfortable in the theatre, I felt bare in the paper scrubs and crocs. I was shivering.

After Surgery, the patient was taken to the recovery room. I watched as Dawn and Sally performed the observations several times every 5 minutes. Dawn explained that as part of the placement I would be concentrating on the 'ABC' assessment criteria, assessing the patient's airway breathing and circulation. Both Dawn and Sally were smiling and calm on the first day, I thought I was going to fit in, I thought I was going to be supported, and I thought it was a great learning opportunity I was wrong.

At the start of my shift with Dawn we read through the list of patients, we would be looking after in the theatre department including a patient undergoing hip surgery and a patient having plastic surgery. Dawn had an image of herself as a 'dynamic nurse teacher,' instead, she was a controlling bully with deep-rooted personal problems.

The sixty-seven-year-old lady, was admitted with hip surgery, and when she was taken into the recovery room, I began the ABC assessment. Dawn had asked me to recite the ABC assessment verbally to her.

"That is not the full assessment try better next time!" she warned.

I felt degraded as she shouted in front of the other staff. Then she explained that we needed to mobilize Betty in the bed to remove the theatre sheets. Dawn could see that I was nervous, and she grabbed my hands to position them onto the patient roughly. "This is the position your hands need to be when you mobilise a patient!" she shouted. I carried on, I should have shouted assault I should have walked out. As a student, you try to put up with your mentor's behaviour, but this behaviour was not acceptable.

In between waiting for the surgery, Dawn would test my knowledge constantly and smile when she caught me out. The questions she asked me were more suitable for junior doctors, I felt like she was trying to catch me out.

"Right the next patient is coming out I need you to be fast and snappy you are too slow!" she growled. Laura came out from her surgery after having full plastic surgery on her face. I felt like I was under police watch, my heart was beating out of my chest. Dawn was standing in front of me, and even without talking I felt uncomfortable around her. The patient was padded up with cotton wool after plastic surgery. Dawn looked at my observations and grabbed the sheet and ripped it up, "Her observations were 19, not 21 I just counted, "she snapped.

"They were 19 when I counted."

"Do not contradict me, I will have to observe you taking observations directly from now on!" she snapped. I felt like I was being contradicted, I was competent in completing observations, and now Dawn was making me doubt my abilities. I felt like a failure.

Before the end of the shift, I watched a right hip replacement and as I observed the surgery, I began to feel very hot and dizzy, and my heart began to race. Then it happened I collapsed onto the floor, I fainted.

I woke up in the recovery room with the monster Dawn looking at me with repulsion.

"Look, I don't want to go into what happened in the theatre I'm already angry with you. Listen, you have a lot of work to do, you will be working with me tomorrow in intensive care, be there at 7 am sharp".

I gulped. I was terrified, a whole day with Dawn on my own spelled nothing but trouble.

The next day as I walked into the intensive care, I could see that we were only looking after one patient who was undergoing chemotherapy treatment. The day in the intensive care unit was like a scene from a horror film. Being alone with Dawn in the room allowed her to treat me in any way she wanted, she constantly tested my knowledge, criticized every task, and even brought a false allegation about me to my university team to assassinate my character. After I completed the shift I vomited outside the hospital, I knew I had failed the placement. I realized how dangerous Dawn was after that shift. I denied the allegation, and subsequently failed the placement. I reported Dawn's behaviour to my university team and submitted an official complaint. I did not let Dawn's behaviour destroy me, all though she had attempted to break me her behaviour made me resilient. I did not learn anything in my theatre placement only the evil nature of human beings. Ever since my negative experience, I always encourage student nurses to speak up about bullying. I left it until the final day of my placement to discuss the bullying and it was too late.

Three months later, I bumped into a Sister in the stroke ward she asked me about my student nurse journey and explained that she had also been a student in the theatre with Dawn.

"I went through horrendous bullying under Dawn she made my life hell. I submitted a complaint. I wish she could see me know she thought that she broke me, but she turned me into a fighter."

Suddenly, I did not feel so alone.

After the theatre placement, I felt like I was standing under a black cloud and needed to pick myself up again. I felt depressed lost and deflated. I was thankful that I had a break from my studies.

When I returned home from London, I went back to my childhood home, I put all my photos in a box and looked over all the stories I had written. Working in the hospital had taken over my entire life, I felt I had no time to complete my work. I looked through all my work I had completed as a teenager, including the war story I wrote as a child, and the fantasy adventures I had written. I still hoped they would be published, and I would achieve my dream to become a successful author.

That afternoon, I went downstairs for my spaghetti meal, and my mother sent me a newspaper clipping, 'missing book found after seven years I looked at the picture in shock, Fernando had returned home, he had been kidnapped seven years ago and was trapped inside an underground farmhouse, and made to work as a slave with several other teenagers. I could not comprehend what happened. I had spent years wondering what happened, I thought he had died, I thought he would never return. The news article explained that the man who kidnapped him, Arnold, worked as a military officer and kidnapped the children to keep him company, and to take care of the crops on the farm. Then as soon as the teenagers grew older, he would kill them. Fernando's successful escape had uncovered the evil truth.

It was now summertime, and one of the hottest summers I had ever experienced. I had so many plans to go to Ireland to visit my family, go to centre parks for the week, and travel to one of my favourite towns Northumberland.

I decided to visit Fernando at his house near the city centre. Fernando lived in a stoned cottage with a picket fence and a swing on the front porch. As I knocked on the door Rita opened the door and began to cry.

"Oh, Mark, it's wonderful to see you again, Fernando will be delighted to see you." She smiled.

I nervously walked into the living room, and I found Fernando sitting in the dining room chair in a white top and grey genes. I felt shocked as I looked at his grey appearance, he was pale, very thin, he had scratches all over his skin, his eyes were filled with tears.

Rita left us alone in the room I was terrified of what he was going to say, so much had changed for me whilst he was trapped in a nightmare.

"It is great to see your mark," it has been seven years since I've seen you- "

"Look we don't need to talk about that now."

"No, we can talk about it," he explained.

I listened in horror as Fernando spoke of the life of slavery, he endured for seven years. Fernando was trapped in the mansion in the cellar with over thirty teenagers. They would spend the days picking the vegetables in the crop field, and cleaning the mansion, with an old flannel and a bucket of water. Fernando stated that the captor Mike would only give the children scrap pieces of bread, and by the end of the week they would congregate in the great hall for a luxury meal on the gigantic dining room table, this was the only luxury they had. Each day, they would all sleep on the cold wooden floorboards resting their heads on each other as their only comfort. Then when one of the teenagers would die, they would bury them under the floorboards. Fernando only escaped when Mike dropped the key on the floor, and he decided to exit on his own, he was traumatized and scared.

It was great to have my old best friend back, but it was clear he was very traumatized by what happened. Over the summer for the first few weeks every Friday, we would go on an hour-long bike ride. On our journey, we would reminisce talking about the past, and occasionally Fernando would talk about his life in the home.

Then at the end of the summer, we planned a trip to Alton towers, the trip we were meant to go on before he was kidnapped. It appeared that

Fernando was doing well, he had put on more weight, took pride in his appearance, and signed up for a college course to finish his A-Levels. During the day we went on the rides, the log flume, the bumper cars, and had a burger meal for lunch. Then the next day when I went to my bank, I found that all my money was gone, Fernando had stolen all my money and disappeared from the town. I never saw Fernando again.

Chapter 8: Summer working have me a blast

Before I commenced my third year of studying, I applied at the nurse bank as a healthcare assistant. I needed to gain confidence after such a negative experience in the theatre. Working as a healthcare assistant improved my communication and clinician skills. Each morning I would be placed in different wards and departments, and it was so challenging working in different wards with different staff and getting used to new routines.

I completed my first shift at a local community hospital in a stroke ward, I was shocked at the lack of security on the wards. Each ward had a green buzzer that automatically opened the door when I was so used to intercoms that opened the door. When I opened the door, I noticed a different setting, as I walked in there was a day room filled with old flowery chairs and a black and white television in the middle of the room. Then outside of the day room where the private rooms where the patients resided. A nurse in pigtails walked up to me smiling,

"Hi what's your name?"

"Hello, I'm Mark."

"Well, Martin you will be looking after patients in rooms one to one with senior nurse Kai and agency nurse Armesh. The patients were on the rehab ward recovering after a stroke. Each patient would have intensive physiotherapy treatment each day. I walked into the first room to help

Arnold a 50-year-old 7-foot man. Kai explained that Arnold had refused to talk since the stroke due to his depression. We used the standing hoist to help Arnold into the shower. Then just as we started to run the water Kai explained that he had to rush off to a ward meeting, leaving the room. There I was suddenly left alone in the shower with a 7-foot patient. How is the possible how could I be left in the room alone? I pressed the buzzer in desperation, and Nurse Richards walked into the room, helping me finish supporting Arnold and then hoisting him into the shower.

After I supported Arnold, I stormed over to Kai in a fit of rage.

"How could you leave me alone with a patient a hoist requires two people!" I shouted.

"How dare you speak to me like that I am a senior nurse!" he roared.

I then assisted Amesha with the next patient Jonathon. Jonathon required full assistance with wash and dressing after he was admitted with a full stroke. I watched Amesha who had an unusual method of washing patients. I watched as he placed the wipes in the bowl and squeezed the water from them.

"This is how you wash a patient; you rinse the cloth until it is bone dry." He warned. I found the people in the shift very difficult to work with.

After washing the patients, we helped to transfer the patients to the day room. I was shocked as the patients sat in front of the television bored and under-stimulated. I decided to administrate puzzles and books to help stimulate the patients, the staff had seemed content for the patients to sit stationary in the room. Suddenly, a confused man Eric stood up with no aids and suddenly he became unsteady. I rushed with Kai to assist the patient to sit on his chair. I was so happy to finish the shift at 1pm.

I then commenced a shift on a specialist dementia unit. A dementia ward that catered for the needs of patients from the early stages of dementia right to the later stages of the illness. The was painted in pale purple calming calls, on the door was a doorbell and a securely locked door requiring key code access. By the nurses' desk was a day room with multiple tables filled with jigsaws, old pictures to encourage reminiscence, and a cassette player to listen to old songs. The red door in the dining room, led to a beautiful garden filled with daffodils roses and a beautiful pond. The ward next to the dementia ward was a general medical ward which some patients would escape to during the shift.

Martina, the ward sister, was dressed in an old-fashioned nurse's outfit to give the feel of an old nurse's outfit and made sure she knew the names of each patient. Bianca and Hayley the ward nurses were able to provide emphatic communication and planned exciting activities for patients.

On my shift, I was looking after five patients at different stages of the condition. The first patient was Deidre an eighty-nine-year-old lady with advanced dementia who enjoyed singing. The second patient was Gill a sixty-year-old lady who developed early-onset dementia which forced her to leave her role. The third patient was Michael an 89-year-old man and former soldier, who believed he was still in the army and would often request order and control on the ward. In the side room was Laurie 90-year-old woman with late-stage dementia who required full support with her dementia condition. In the fifth bed was Daniel, a forty-year-old man, who had been diagnosed with frontal temporal dementia, and was struggling to come to terms with his condition.

Each patient was going through their journey and I was so happy to help each patient.

I enjoyed supporting Deirdre she would sing random songs and in the middle of the ward, she led me into the waltz for the song let us face the music, and dance after I helped her with her wash and dressing room. In the dayroom, she watched her favourite film, 'The wizard of oz, and as she sang 'somewhere over the rainbow' three other patients sat beside her holding her hand joining in with the words in unison. In the afternoon when it started raining, Deidre demanded to go outside and began to dance in the rain singing, 'singing in the rain,' dancing in a choreographed way. It was no surprise to me that Deidre was a former actress on Broadway. In the late afternoon, Deidre had managed to slip away from the ward and into the next ward. We looked on in shock as she lay in the same bed as an eighty-year-old man who was asleep in the bed. I slowly walked up to her in the bed and tapped her on the shoulder. Suddenly, Deidre burst out of the bed singing 'under the boardwalk' and I walked with her to the other ward.

Gill struggled to accept her diagnosis having to leave work and come to terms with the illness on her phone, following the breakdown of her marriage. Gill wore a black business suit and would constantly write down facts and encourage staff to write down events of the day.

In Gills room were so many lists, lists of her clothes that she brought in, and lists of the dates of all her children's birthdays.

"Oh, Mark can you help me? I want you to write a list of today's events just so I can be sure of what we are doing,"

"Of course, I can," I smiled. I wrote down a timetable for the day. I tried to initiate Gill to come to the day room to take part in the activities, but she wanted to stay in her room. On her bedside table, Gill had a scrapbook of photos from her forty-year teaching career, and a tablet that displayed photos and videos from key parts of her life.

Throughout the day, Gill would stay in her side room constantly scribbling notes in her side room, even writing her memories in a reflective memoir for condition progressed. The nurses had to decide if

Gill was more suited to staying at home or residing in a specialist unit for people living with dementia.

I supported Laurie in the side room, Laurie was living with end-stage dementia. Laurie was 85 years old and was surrounded by daffodils and roses. Laurie was a church vicar, and a dozen cards were hanging on a string in the room. As a team, we supported Laurie with her care, and she required full assistance with feeding. Laurie's little compact radio played her favourite songs from Elvis to Frank Sinatra. As the music played Laurie reached for my hand and moved it in motion to the music. It was so rewarding supporting Laurie and it was the true essence of nursing care, being there door a patient at their most vulnerable. Holding a person's hand was all Laurie needed to feel secure.

In the main bay was Michael, a 99-year-old ex-soldier. Michael had figures of soldiers lined up on his table. During the shift, Michael would fold his clothes and bedsheets. Michael was so used to order and structure that he carried it over to every part of his life. In the day room, the staff, Marina, Bianca, and Hayley encouraged everyone to stand in a line and repeat our names. Michael would watch in awe and at times he still believed he was in the army. The ward staff was conscientious in supporting the needs of each patient, and on national Memorial Day they played patriotic songs, and decorated the table with a patriotic flag, the staff supported each patient with their needs.

In the final side room was Dan, a forty-two-year-old man who had been diagnosed with frontal temporal dementia, and he was displaying more confusion after a refusal to take tablets. Dan's wife had reached crisis point, and called the ambulance team when he was caught sitting on a window ledge. Dan was distraught after losing his job as a builder which he did for over 26 years. During Dan's day, he was very tearful about his condition. I had the time to talk to him to remind him of the importance of seeing his friends, taking part in exercise, and keeping his mind stimulated. I sat beside Dan and made a note of local groups and services that can support him and improve the quality of his life.

I enjoyed the shift on the dementia ward. I had worked so often on wards in which patients with dementia were constricted on generic wards and were prohibited from completing day-to-day activities. It was wonderful to watch patients moving around, freely, and being able to choose the activities they want to do. Staff had time to sit with patients, and offer the specialized support they needed.

I started a nightshift at the general medical ward with my nightshift survival bag in my hand. In my nightshift bag, I had several bags of crisps a fizzy drink, and a toothbrush. It was always difficult starting a night shift on a new ward, there was a fear of being moved to a different department and of not fitting in with the team.

As I walked into the ward Leanne the lead nurse advised me that I would be supporting a patient in the side room by offering one-to-one support. I was joined by nurse Emily and health care assistant Becky on the ward.

"Hello, Mark if you need help please just ask. The patient John had been admitted for total hip surgery but was now experiencing acute delirium in his recovery. As I walked into the side room, I could see John sitting up in his bed looking anxious. John had long grey wispy hair and wore blue chequered panamas.

"Who are you? I just got rid of one nurse!" He moaned.

"I'm Mark, I'm here to look after you tonight."

I watched as John appeared to roll his eyes in frustration, as he sat calmly in his bed reading. I had looked after patients who had experienced delirium previously. Delirium would often make patients act out of character, such as shouting out, becoming increasingly aggressive, and slurring their speech.

An hour into the shift John jumped up from his bed, "right I need to go now, I have had enough, He exclaimed, grabbing his stick.

John then left the side room and appeared to walk up and down the ward trying to find an exit.

I watched as the nurses Leanne, Emily, and the healthcare assistant Becky sat at the nurse station devouring their donuts and crisps.

"Good luck darling we are here if you need us," Leanne smiled whilst taking a bite of her donut.

John's breathing became heavier, and he charged out of the ward and walked over to the orthopaedic ward.

"John, we need to go back to our ward," I warned.

"Shut up Pinocchio, I need to go home," John shouted.

John pushed through the double doors and into the orthopaedic ward. The ward staff looked startled as John walked into the main bay, sitting on the bed of a sleeping female patient. The patient jumped up and looked on in shock.

"who on earth are you? Get off my bed!" she warned.

"I'm so sorry," I exclaimed.

I looked on at John who gave an emotionless expression and refused to move.

"Please John can you get off the bed you are disturbing the patient?" I requested.

The ward had called the security, but it did not seem to deter John. Ten minutes later, John charged along the corridor of the ward grabbing the fire extinguisher. Jon stood outside the fire extinguisher and stood by the door.

"Right one of you open the door now," he warned.

"No, we cannot open the door it leads to the edge of a cliff," warned Simon the security guard.

"Right, I will count to ten and if you do not open the door, I will break it open," He shouted.

John counted down from ten and he broke down the door in anger. I watched as the security guards guided him back to the medical ward, explaining it was a place to go 'home,' When I returned to the medical ward the witches of Eastwick continued to sit at the desk tucking into their snacks.

"well done your doing an amazing job!" Emily scoffed.

As I guided John back to the side room, he appeared more relaxed. John sat in his armchair, and began to tell me about his life as a truck driver. As John explained that he picked up a hitch hiker and crashed into a bush, I began to laugh and suddenly Mike grabbed his jug of water and thew it at me and it narrowly missed me, John then proceeded to grab his table and in deep anger, he snapped the table in two.

John then stomped out of the room, and began to look around the ward mischievously, he reached the store cupboard where he found a bag of tennis balls and to the surprise of Leanne Emily and Becky, he began to throw the tennis balls at them, disturbing them from their peaceful night. I watched as they jumped up, horrified, and angry, trying desperately to catch the balls,

"Mark! Don't just stand there stop John!" Leanne warned. After John had finished throwing the thirty balls, I helped to guide him to the bed, and he dived under the covers and fell into a deep sleep. It was now 6 am, I was exhausted, I did not have time to sit down or have a break all night. Working a night shift and providing one-to-one care to a confused patient was both mentally and physically draining. It was now the end of my summer job, but I was to take one final trip before I commenced the third year.

Before I commenced third year, Mike had revealed that his Father had won ten million pounds. As a surprise for us, Mike had booked for us all to travel to Florida with him for two weeks. It was the break that I needed after such a tough year. We were all so excited for the break it was a dream getaway. On the eleven-hour flight, I watched my favourite films Titanic and avatar. Mike and John were singing their favourite records whilst drinking alcohol. Laura sat by the window reading her collection of books, and Martha sat with her face mask on sipping on her ice lemonade.

We arrived at a beautiful villa with a swirl pool, three Jacuzzi's, a games room and ten bedrooms. As we entered the apartment, John, Mike, and Martha dived into the pool. Whist I collapsed onto the sofa I was exhausted.

It was a magical journey throughout the two weeks. On our first morning, we went to the Hollywood walk of the frame and put our hands to the imprints before heading into the town with our chocolate ice creams.

We had an amazing time at Disney World in Florida, John and Mike proceeded to run off together on their own in an attempt to go on every single ride. I was stuck with Martha for the day, on each right she proceeded to scream at the top of her lungs it was deafening. Martha dragged me to each shop, filling her bag with souvenirs and Disney clothes, I had to carry five bags filled with Disney memorabilia.

Laura proceeded to spend the whole day sitting on a bench reading her Danielle Steele books, she was the only person I knew who would go to a theme park and read books all day.

Each day over the two weeks we would go to the theme parks and sightseeing, we would relax at night by the poolside listening to our favourite songs, and watching films on the widescreen television.

On the final day of our holiday, as both I and Martha were walking into the town after visiting the Hollywood sign, we bumped into a mysterious fortune teller, who guided us into a tent for reading. I was reluctant to engage but Martha explained that I just had to go with her.

The fortune-teller explained to me that my current role as a student nurse was temporary, and that my career as a nurse was temporary, and that I was to partake in many different careers.

The fortune-teller warned Martha that she needs to seek support before her personal traumatic experiences, she warned Martha that she needed to seek help before it was too late. In a state of terror, Martha ran out of the tent in tears. If only I had listened if only Martha had listened to the fortune teller our futures would have taken a different turn.

Chapter 9: Final year: The cardiac ward

I started the final year of my course and was excited to be starting on a cardiac ward. I was born with a heart murmur, and spent many times in my life, going to cardiac appointments, and had a personal interest in the cardiology field. My confidence was at rock bottom following the theatre placement, and I was about to enter award in which I would receive extensive support from all ward staff in helping me to achieve my outcomes.

The cardiology ward was a busy 30 bedded ward, the patients were admitted for minor cardiac complaints, whilst others were admitted for cardiac surgery, and like most medical ward's patients were also admitted with general medical concerns.

I was so nervous on my first day, as a student nurse in the final year, I had to now prove that I was competent in completing nursing competencies. My mentor on the ward was sister Jenny, an experienced nurse from Ireland, who nursed for over forty years. Siter Jenny was kind, approachable, and strived to support final year students and mentored newly qualified nurses. Holly the health care assistant I would work alongside, was very lazy, and spent most of her time sitting on a chair, taking pictures of herself, or face timing her boyfriend in London. Nurse Rita was an experienced nurse practitioner, with over twenty years of experience as a nurse. Rita was able to give a clinical explanation for all nursing observations.

Nurse Sharmaine was a sarcastic nurse, and proceeded to call me Tony, she was also clumsy and would often fall and trip over work surfaces. The cardiology ward was welcoming, and all the staff was smiling, relaxed and content on the ward. I was so happy to work in such a calm supportive environment.

From the moment I entered the ward, I could hear the beeping of the cardiac monitors, and the sounds of the observation machines taking their current readings.

On my first shift, I was looking after four patients in the bay and two patients in the side room. In the side room was Edward a 102-year-old man, and previous soldier, admitted from a care home with worsening symptoms in his dementia. In the second side room was Gill, a nighty eight-year-old lady recovering from stent surgery.

In the bay was Debra, a lady admitted with worsening mobility coinciding with her vascular dementia.

Next to Debra, was Deidre, an eighty-year-old lady requiring one-to-one mental health support after refusing to take her medication for her bipolar disorder. Deidre was supported by a mental health nurse at all times. Opposite Deidre was Gemma, an eighty-nine-year-old lady admitted with recurrent urinary tract infections and complained constantly about the noise in the ward.

Then next to Gemma was Laura, who was recovering from her triple bypass surgery and required consistent support with going to the toilet.

At the start of the shift, after the drug round Sister Jenny, Holly and Sharmaine joined as a team to help wash the patients together.

I spent the time supporting Edward and Gill in the side room. Edward had pictures in his room of his time as a general in the army. Every time I attempted to ask Edward about his army days, he stated 'It was none of my business,' Edward appeared relaxed in his bed covered in ten blankets. Edward was awake all night on the ward and violently tried to escape by breaking the door with his walking stick and began to sing-song at the top of his lung, waking all of the patients on the ward. On the day shift, he appeared to recover from his night before.

I supported Gill with mobilizing into her chair, as she had become quite weak after her surgery. Gill sat quietly knitting in her chair recalling her time as a tonalist during the war following the death of her husband. Gill was able to recall her fight for women's rights, attending various marches in London, and giving speeches on the plea for equal rights.

After all the patients were washed and dressed, I had to carefully decide the treatment plans for each patient. I was suddenly met with so many challenges in my bay. Debra became increasingly confused, and began to crawl around the floor even though she could walk.

"Debra why are you crawling, it would be better and safer if you could walk on the ward."

"No, I can't it's not safe I could drown.'

Due to Debra's dementia, the colours of the floor led to her confusion as the blue circles around the orange painted floor made her feel unsafe. I assigned photo queen Holly to provide one-to-one support to Debra.

I took Deidre's observations and she sat colouring in her book. I could see how agitated Deidre was constantly fidgeting and being unable to sit still in her seat.

As Deidre sat in the armchair, I explained that she was going to be transferred to the Mars Centre for furfur assessment of her mental health needs. As soon as I announced her transfer Deidre began to fly off into a fit of rage.

"How can I be persecuted like this? My husband has full custody of my child I am trying desperately to fight for visitation, and I'm being sent away!"

"You are going to get help at the Mars centre," stated Stacey the mental health nurse.

"I've had just about enough of you, just shit up your fat bitch," she roared, throwing her cold jug of water at the poor nurse. It was clear to see that Diedre was very stressed, and I pushed for an earlier discharge due to her distress.

Gemma called me over in anger, "Nurse move me out of this mad room, I want to go into the side room it is too noisy I hate it out here!" she whined.

"I will try my best to get you into the side room,"

"Well try a bit harder!" she roared.

Laura clicked her fingers at me, I assisted her to the toilet whilst carrying her drip-feed behind her.

When I returned to the bay, I had to complete all the end of bed notes, making sure the skin charts were filled in, and that the patient's fluid and dietary intake was filled in quietly. I felt under pressure already knowing that Deidre and Debra required extra support this made it difficult to provide full support to the other patients. Holly persisted for Debra to stand, but she continued to crawl over the floor, whilst the mental health nurse maintained an adequate distance from Deidre and herself.

Jenny had asked me to help her complete the discharge notes for Gemma and Laura and in the distance, I could see Holly taking pictures of herself in the distance.

I was incredibly nervous on my first day still, I felt like I was in a goldfish bowl. As we completed the checklist the porters arrived to help transfer Diedre to the mental health assessment unit. As the porters arrived Deidre let out a scream.

"Deidre, whatever is the matter?"

"I'm not going until I have a bible in front of me and you can swear that I will go home one day." She warned.

Jenny passed her a green bible from the cupboard, but she stated a true bible would never be green. In a state of anger Gemma grabbed a blue bible and threw it on Deidre's bed, "Take the bible and get the hell out of here we are sick of you!" she shouted.

Jenny promised Deidre that the staff at the assessment centre would try their best to help her prepare to go home, and thankfully Deidre left and she was discharged.

I had to be very methodical in my thinking remembering when observations were to be completed, checking when medications were to be completed, and completing all the dressings.

As I completed the observations, Jenny explained her difficult road to being a nurse. Jenny moved to Birmingham at twenty years of age the oldest of ten siblings. Jenny's parents had both passed away leaving her alone to raise her siblings. Jenny trained at the local hospital during the night, and worked the night shift five days a week, with her young brother, at a local food warehouse trying desperately to survive.

After I completed the observations, Gill called me into the side room, and explained that she was terrified of leaving the ward at 102 she wanted company, she offered to volunteer at the hospital, after she left to help keep her stimulated. I referred Gill to the local Age UK community group, to get her to meet other people and decrease her loneliness.

I felt that working on the ward helped already to build my confidence. The staff was always on hand to support, and Sister Jenny allowed me to learn in a relaxed way, through answering questions, and trying new skills whilst teaching me the evidence base behind nursing procedures.

After 5 pm, a new patient was admitted into the ward Rita Bartholomew from India, Rita could not speak English, Rita's daughter Shelly translated everything she said to the team. Rita had been admitted after having a panic attack. As soon as I introduced myself Rita began to speak in her own language, fast, I asked the daughter what she was saying.

"Mother thinks that you are a nice young boy, but she would prefer a female nurse." I watched as Rita began to cry hysterically and held her hands on her head looking on helplessly.

"Mum stated she is so upset and wants you to send her to a side room because she feels it is too noisy," she whined. It was common for a male student nurse to have female patients refuse treatment.

I had been able to complete the observations, dressings, and nursing notes in time. Before the end of the first shift, Richard had pressed his buzzer for assistance.

When I walked in, I could see him laying in his bed reading his war book.

"Please sire can I have five blankets I'm feeling cold?" He explained. I grabbed the blankets from the cupboard and helped to position Richard in the bed, as his head hit the pillow, he began to make exaggerated snoring noises and I felt like he was settled for the night.

Two minutes later, as I assisted Laura to the bathroom, I could hear a banging noise in the distance. As I walked to the empty G bay, I witnessed Richard trying to break the fire door exit with his walking stick. This was the nature of nursing; you can never predict what can happen in a matter of minutes.

Chapter 10: The lift of terror

Throughout the cardiology placement, I felt fully supported by all staff members. I enjoyed my nursing course again, I felt like I was at rock bottom at the theatre placement, and I was now feeling content in my abilities.

It was the morning of my 23rd birthday, it was always difficult to spend your birthday on a ward for twelve hours, so I was already in a sombre mood. I went into the lift hoping to get to the third floor for the cardiology ward. As the ward travelled up it bolted with a sudden spark, and I knew instantly we were trapped. In the bay was Greg the hospital porter holding the patient wheelchair which Rex sat in. At 95, Rex was living with dementia, and held onto his stick aggressively. In the corner of the lift opposite me was Nurse Jill who was already nervous and scared. Next to Lexi, was Dawn, a confused patient who wore bright pink pyjamas and was smelling of smoke from a smoking trip outside.

"Don't worry we will be out before you know it this has happened before!" Greg stammered.

"We have to get out soon I have an appraisal meeting with my manager it is serious," Lexi shouted. I then observed Rex using his stick to lift Lexi's skirt.

"Do you mind? she shouted.

"well, you have to try your luck at any opportunity!" he shouted.

We had only been in the lift for ten minutes and it was too long.

Greg picked up an alert on his phone and explained that he had sent a text to the maintenance team.

"The team will be working on getting us back as soon as possible," Greg warned.

Everyone appeared to be relaxed, while we waited anxiously for the team. We were all concerned about Dawn's erratic behaviour and she began to pace back and forth, then suddenly she erupted at me.

"Why can't we get out? I need a smoke!" She shouted.

"We are stuck we just have to wait it won't be long now," I promised,

"If you don't open the door now, I am going to scream," she warned.

Suddenly Dawn erupted into a tremendous fit of rage and began to smack the doors of her lift with her fists.

I leaned down on the floor, trying to relax, we waited and waited but the maintenance team was delayed. It was now three hours. We could finally hear the noise of the maintenance team coming through Greg's intercom.

"Don't worry we will get you out soon," boomed the calming voice.

Then suddenly the lift bolted, and it began to drop and then the lift crashed, and the lights went out. We were now in pitch black.

"That sounds bad," I warned.

"Fucking hell! Let me out of this lift now I can't cope with you, inbred bastards!" Dawn shouted. I could then hear Dawn charge forward towards Rex and she tried desperately to grab his stick.

"Give me your Stick I need to break the door down."

"Let it go your fat cow!" Rex shouted, before hitting out with his stick whacking me in the arm, before hitting Dawn, causing her to collapse onto the floor in terror whilst Lexi comforted her.

As Time was going by tensions began to grow, and Rex stood up and began to urinate on the floor. After a few hours both Dawn and Rex had collapsed on the floor, into a deep sleep after eight hours the maintenance team managed to help get us out. I was exhausted, Sister Jenny allowed me to go home, and I collapsed into my bed hysterically crying. It was one of the most traumatic events of my life and I will never forget it. That weekend after the lift incident my life was about to be turned upside down.

My parents explained that they were leaving, and they wanted me to collect my things and help to bring the boxes out of the lift and help to put them on the truck. I was searching through the boxes many of my old clothes, toys, and sentimental pictures were packed in boxes. Then under an old broken Christmas tree, I found a red sealed box with the word, 'Do not open on the lid.

I could not help it I had to see what was inside. I opened the box and inside was a birth certificate and an adoption certificate. It was my certificate; I had just discovered I was adopted at the age of twenty-three. In the box were the name and address of my biological parents. I collapsed into a heap, I was shocked, scared, angry, and filled with terror. I could not move I was numb.

"Mark hurry up," Mum shouted.

I quickly sealed the contents in the box, I could not let anyone know that I knew the truth. I exited the loft and caught a train to London. I managed to track down the address of my biological parents, Kate and Michael in Buckinghamshire, they lived in a beautiful three-story Edwardian mansion. I arrived early at the house at 7 am early in morning, a delivery truck arrived outside. As the delivery driver exited with the box, I lied, saying that I lived in the house and he passed me the box. I knocked on the door shaking, and then my mother Kate opened the door. Kate stood wearing a bright blue dress with pink glassed wearing a diamond necklace. In the distance, I could see my father sitting on a chair reading the times. I wanted to blurt out that they were my parents I wanted to ask why they had abandoned me.

"Hi, I've come to drop off a parcel to you, I live around the corner," I exclaimed.

"Oh, that's kind of you, I must tell the royal mail not to leave my mail with strangers in the future. This is a disgrace!" she moaned, before slamming the door.

That was the closure I needed, I was an adult, my parents at my family home, where my real parents loved and cared for me. I decided to keep that day a secret, I did not reveal my newfound knowledge to my parents until three years later. I tried so hard to block it out and working as a student nurse and focusing on my course helped to block it out.

Chapter 11: Accident and Emergency.

The two years of my course seemed to go so quickly, and I had packed so much into my course. I had worked in a range of settings including a stroke ward, a district nursing placement, and a palliative care ward. It was rewarding watching patients improve and successfully overcome their illnesses. It also felt rewarding to support patients in the final stages of their condition.

I was coming to the final stage of my course, and was now on my final placement as a student nurse. I was working on a busy accident and emergency ward and had supported patients who had been involved in roadside accidents, minor injuries and supported patients of a wide age range from children to adults. My mentor Judith had over thirty years of experience as a senior nurse on accident and emergency and was also a student coordinator.

At the flat we were all coping with the sudden loss of Martha, Martha had struggled to find acting work following a successful stint in completing commercials, and a successful run-in west end in the wicked play.

Martha had jumped off a cliff in Colorado, leaving a suicide note explaining she could no longer go on anymore.

The atmosphere in the flat was so difficult without Martha she was the life of the party. As a group, it felt like we were all moving in different directions. Laura was finishing her medical studies and would soon be leaving, John was getting ready to marry his fiancé and move into his new home in Essex, whilst Mike continued to live in the flat singing in different pubs and restaurants.

Each morning, before a shift, I would consume my warm bowl of porridge with my freezing orange juice. Then I would set out on the cobbled path at 6:00 am and arrived at the ward at 6:30 am. I walked into the ward which had the desk in the centre with the trolley beds situated around the desk in a circular pattern. There were only five patients in the bay, which was unusual for the morning. I observed the staff I would be working with, including Kelly, a very abrupt young nurse who was a mentor to Ann a twenty-year-old student in her second-year placement, and struggled working alongside Kelly's defiant attitude. Tara was a healthcare assistant, with over twenty years of experience working in the hospital, and could complete advanced clinical duties.

I had learned so much from Juliet in my placement and today was my final placement. I had learned how to respond to emergencies, how to clinically support a deteriorating patient, I also learned how to manage a ward in preparation for being a nurse.

In the handover, I was assigned five patients in cubicle A who had just been admitted. The first patient was Rick a twenty-eight-year-old man admitted with deep wounds, following a fight in prison he was admitted in cuffs with prison guards for supervision.

Simon was admitted at 100 years of age, with shortness of breath, and was now a renowned war veteran.

Then in cubicle 3 was John admitted following a worsening in his dementia condition, setting fire to the kitchen, and his wife being unable to cope.

In Cubicle 4 was Hayley a thirty-five-year-old woman, angry, waiting for her medication following being admitted with complications in her asthma condition.

In cubicle 5 was Mena an eighty-one-year-old lady from Bulgaria admitted with diarrhoea and vomiting and consigned to the side room.

I was nervous attending to the first patient Rick, especially after hearing about his violent and angry temperament. As I walked up to him, I observed the aggressive look on his face, with the words 'fuck you' tattooed on his neck I was not holding out for a pleasant conversation. I prepared the nursing trolley to apply the dressing on his leg. As I began to wipe his wounded leg, I looked at the terror on his face.

"You're too rough you are fucking bastard." He shouted.

"I'm sorry I'm nearly there I promised,"

"You're too slow your stupid bastard!" he growled, before spitting at me, as I managed to carefully apply the dressing. It was difficult supporting patients who were aggressive, but as a nurse, you have a duty of care to support all patients. I watched as he shot back an angry expression, I was glad he would be going home early in the morning.

I observed Juliet rushing around completing notes and answering all the never-ending phone calls at the nurse's station, but I knew she was always there for me if I needed her.

I then went to support Simon who was admitted with Shortness of breath and he had just finished his nebulizer.

"How are you feeling? I understand you came here in quite a panic last night?

"Yes, it's difficult, it is hard living without my wife we were together for seventy years and I guess I am struggling without her." He explained.

"How do you feel you are managing at home? Do you feel you need any assistance?"

"I'm feeling so depressed, I could do with a cleaner, I'm also finding it hard completing wash and dressing activities, I need a little bit of help," he admitted crying. I then raised John's current circumstances with social services, in the hope that he would be able to get help to support him. We later discovered that John had been living alone in his house, for over two years, and his house was swarmed with rats and litter.

I observed Hayley furiously pressing her buzzer, "excuse me nurse how long will it take for my tablets to be ready?" I asked.

"We are just waiting for the pharmacist to sign off the medication, it should be with you shortly," I assured.

"I can't wait too long I have a beauty business; I have to pick up my son from University, then I have the grocery shopping," She added.

"Look, Hayley, I will try my best to speed up the process," I promised.

"Well, if it takes any longer, I will submit a formal complaint!" Hayley warned.

I then walked over to John and completed his observations. John was very tearful. "I want to go home my mother will be expecting me," he cried.

"you just have to stay here a little longer, we just want to make sure that you are well enough."

"It's so noisy here and the train never arrives. What's going on?" he roared. John believed that he was at a train station and became more confused indicating that his dementia condition had worsened. I was very fortunate in the hospital to be supported by a dementia team, who were able to come and sir with John and provide him with purposeful activities.

I then walked over to drink my cut of tea made me the ward clerk, I felt guilt at the nurse station taking a drink, there were always tasks to complete and I almost felt guilty taking a rest break.

I then went to check on Mena in the side room and to my shock, she was laying on the cold hospital floor in her red gown. I alerted Juliet to come and help me, and Mena looked up at me helplessly. "I have not fallen, I am just sitting here helplessly, I just want to go home.

"Oh, Mena, we need to get you up, you can't stay on the floor Mena," I warned. I watched as Mena grabbed the walking frame and she struggled but stood up walked towards her bedside table. As she sat down, she grabbed me and Juliet by the head kissing us wetly as I looked on in terror.

It was already such a busy morning, as stressful as accident and emergency where it was always full of exciting opportunities. As I walked out on the ward, I observed a frustrated Ann sitting in the nurse's office looking stressed, with tears in her eyes.

"What's wrong Ann?" I asked.

"My mentor has only given me two weeks to pass the placement, I can't fail if I fail this course, my dream will be ruined, and I won't be able to stay in my accommodation, and I'm a struggling single mother," she snapped.

"I will meet you at lunchtime at 1 pm we will go through your targets together," I promised. I knew how difficult was to have a difficult mentor and wanted to support Ann as best as I could.

I was nervous halfway through the shift when the ward manager, Jessica, called me into the office. I was delighted to find that Jessica had offered me a job position to start in the following September. I felt that I had finally achieved success after two years of hard work.

When I returned to the ward Rick was now discharged, Simon was asleep, John was completing a jigsaw puzzle with the dementia support walker. Hayley continued to look at us with daggers.

Mena's daughter Brielle called me and Juliet into the side room, "I want to talk to you, I am very disappointed in the both of you!" she roared. When we walked into the side room, we found Mena fast asleep in the bed.

"I want to ask why you both carried my mother into bed?"

"We did not carry her; she used the frame," I added.

"It is not possible to carry your mother into bed she is a lot bigger than the both of us," Juliet added.

"My mother has not walked in over forty years, you are lying!" she roared stamping her feet.

"You did, you carried me into bed," Mena added. We both looked at each other in disbelief, then when we observed Mena's notes, which detailed that she had put in several unsuccessful compensation reports, over twenty years in hospitals and none had been successful.

Suddenly we were called into cubicle ten to help Ann and Kelly with their new patient. The patient was having a seizure and foaming at the mouth and we helped to turn him on his side.

The senior consultant doctor Rhodes rushed in, "tell me about George I have heard he has taken a substance."

"Yes ecstasy, at a party, he is eighteen. He went home following the party and his mother found him lying on the floor."

"Right close the curtain- "

It was then that we heard the emergency buzzer ring with red lights flashing. It was a twenty-year-old man who had collapsed in a nearby football patch. He was admitted with chest pain but became unresponsive and the staff had begun to complete CPR. I watched as the nurses and doctors crowded around the bed, each taking in turns to complete the CPR. I watched as Ann completed the compressions, her face sweating, she was nervous and scared.

It was then that Dr. Roberts ordered me to complete the compression, I could feel my heart pound against my chest as I completed the compressions, and felt the rush of adrenaline, as the senior consultant advised me to go slower than faster. After thirty compressions, I placed the non-breath mouth on Sean before giving mouth to mouth.

Unfortunately, our efforts to save Sean were unsuccessful and he passed away. It was shocking to watch the death of the young twenty-five-year-old man, and it showed the unpredictable nature of working in accident and emergency.

At the end of the shift, Juliet had passed me a box filled with thank you cards and boxes of chocolates and my book, confirming I had passed. I was so happy that I passed after an intensive two years it felt great to finally have direction and a future.

That evening, when I returned home my flatmates were in the dining room eating a roast dinner celebrating the memory of Martha. I decided I could not say goodbye to my flatmates, I wanted to get away, I missed my family and life in Birmingham.

Chapter 12: Casualty

After an eventful six weeks off for the summer, it was time for me to return to work. I decided not to take the accident and emergency job and instead applied for a job on a stroke ward I worked on as a student. The stroke would be filled with dynamic and hardworking staff. Sister Diana who worked as the lead sister, was the most compassionate nurse, I had ever worked with, knowing the names of all the patients providing patient-centred care. Nurse Elsa, was one of the funniest nurses I had ever worked with, and we would constantly hear her sing and dancing putting on a show for the patients. Whilst the manager Rachel was strict and eccentric.

I had spent three weeks working on the ward working supernumerary working as a health care assistant whilst observing the practice of Sister Diana who was helping to prepare for the nursing role.

In my first role in practice, I was supporting five male patients in a bay and two patients in the side room. In Bay A I was looking after Aknesh an 88-year-old man who was living with dementia and Parkinson's disease. Aknesh was admitted with a query stroke and worsening behaviour. The second patient was Bill a forty-two-year-old patient who collapsed at work after suffering from a full stroke. Bill was devastated at the thought of not being able to work and the thought of being permanently disabled for life.

The third patient was nighty one year Tom, who was admitted from a worsening in his dementia condition, admitted from the care home after they struggled to manage.

The fourth patient was Chris, a forty-year-old man, living with the effects of a left-sided stroke and coming to terms with his heroin drug addiction.

The fifth patient, Arnold, a nighty seven-year-old man who fought in the first world war, was very aggressive and was admitted for an assessment of his care needs. In the side room, was a patient called Bill, who was admitted following a right-side stroke. The patient in the second side room was Laura 89-year-old woman with worsening confusion after being diagnosed with mixed dementia.

After the handover, we could hear a loud thud in the side room. We all rushed out and we observed Bill inside room one had fallen from the bed onto the floor. Immediately, I put a pillow under his head, and we helped to hoist him back into the bed. Once Bill was in the bed, I took his blood pressure and took his observations which were all in the normal range, before arranging for a doctor to check him over. I was concerned having just had an emergency in the first minute of my shift.

I took a deep breath and walked into my bay. I was finally the nurse with the name tag on my collar. I was working with the healthcare assistant Alina who was checking the charts. Alina was a chronic smoker who would constantly leave the ward to smoke, I observed her hair steaming in smoke frequently. Most of my patients were asleep, four out of the seven patients I was looking for was living with dementia. This was common in hospitals which did not always cater to the needs of people living with dementia.

I was nervous administrating the tablets on my own and feeling the weight of responsibility on my shoulders.

It was so difficult giving tablets to people living with dementia. As soon as I positioned Aknesh in the bed he grabbed the tablets in the pot and began to crush them. I then walked over to Arnold who stood holding his stick across his chest. "Go away I don't like you I've never liked you!" he roared. I then encouraged Alina to help with the medications as he appeared calmer among the female workers, I watched how calm Arnold was around Alina in stark contrast to how he treated me.

Washing patients on the stroke ward was a big part of the daily routine. Washing and mobilizing patients into the chair into the morning helped to work active movement in the muscles.

I was thankful that Sister Diana was willing to help me wash the patients, whilst Alina washed the other patients but would constantly leave the ward to have her one hundred cigarettes.

The first patient we watched was Aknesh, Aknesh allowed us to support him to start with washing him at the bedside, he appeared calmer following his medication. Then as he sat in the chair he grabbed onto my hand and began to squeeze my fingers before twisting them.

"Oh, Aknesh please let go of my fingers!" I yelled.

Sister Diana shouted for help, and I watched as the physiotherapists' Mat and Daniel came to the rescue. I felt like my fingers were about to break, and it took six members of staff to help Aknesha gently remove his fingers from my hand. I wanted to appear as an in-control newly qualified nurse, but I felt I was drowning.

Then Sister Di and I took on the ultimate challenge and assisted Arnold to the shower room for his wash. I watched as Sister Di linked onto Arnold's arm, she had such a gentle way with the patients, and I watched as they walked together.

"Arnold we are going on a little mission, we are going into the shower, and I want to talk about your stories of your time as a soldier." I assisted

Diana in helping Arnold into the shower and he looked at me with a glare in his eye as he began it sit on the shower stool.

"who the bloody hell is he?" he roared.

"This is Mark he is here to help you," Diana answered.

"What regiment does he belong to?"

"The 7th Brigade," Sister Di responded.

Arnold believed that he was a soldier and any noise sound or object on the ward could resonate with a memory he had in the army. As Diana began to wash him using the shower head, I stepped forward and assisted Arnold with the shower. He turned around and looked at me in anger.

"You Bastard!" he shouted. Arnold proceeded to grab the shower head and began to soak me and hot me across the chest.

Sister Di burst into a fit of laughter as she was able to help him regain his composure.

We then proceeded to wash Chris, Chris was in a deep state of depression as the stroke and the heroin addiction he continued to live with had a deep impact upon him. Chris required full assistance with the wash and required a hoist to get into the chair. It was so difficult to try to motivate patients when they were so low in mood, we could only refer patients to counselling or talking therapies but there was no assurance that patients could take up help.

It was then that Doctor Anila walked onto the ward, dressed in a biker outfit. Doctor Alina was eccentric and would often wear bizarre and outrageous clothes. As soon as Doctor Alina came into the bay, she quickly barked orders for me to complete. I had to complete a dressing for Aknesha, encourage Bill to engage in physio input, and book a mental health assessment for Tom and plan discharge for Lauren and Bill in the side rooms.

After the ward round, I witnessed Aline walking towards the door ready to go out for her one of many cigarettes, I felt a fuse go in my head. "Alina, I need help with the patients we need to complete out turns," I warned.

"Why are you going on at me in the morning and so early? How could you deny me a cigarette? I work so hard; it is not fair!" she screeched. Alina was a formidable force.

I then observed Bill crying by his bedside table, for people living with a stroke it was very emotionally draining and hard to accept being unable to do daily tasks.

"I'm finding it so hard, some days I'm struggling to speak, I have to have help to eat, I have to have help to move. I will never be able to work again." He cried hysterically.

"You can do it, you must remain positive, you have to engage in therapy, you have to make an effort," I assured him.

When Mat and John the physiotherapists came to the bedside, they stood at wither side of Bill and they encouraged him to stand by first completing bed exercises, then Mat put a walking frame in front of Bill and within minutes he stood. I watched as tears rolled down Bill's face, the look of desperation on his face now turned to disbelief and happiness. Bill was ecstatic that he could finally mobilize, it was an emotional time.

As the physiotherapists moved Bill to the physio treatment for further therapy, I looked around my bay and noticed a rare moment of calmness, families had started to arrive and the patients were sitting out into their chairs, calm and composed.

As I walked out of the bay, I noticed Nurse Elsa in bay c, all her patients were calm, and I noticed her dancing to 9-5 with her patient. "Oh Mark, please can you make me a cup of tea, I'm exhausted!" she shouted.

As soon as I walked over to the nurse's station the ward Clark Dora provided me with a dozen messages, explaining I had to contact several family members, complete discharge letters, and contact various members of the multidisciplinary team. I felt like I had no free time as a nurse, I was constantly busy and would even feel guilty for sitting down for two minutes. As I stood at the desk, Sister Diana passed me a warm cup of tea and a biscuit. "Well done Mark you are doing well," she assured. Sister Diana was positive and would always make staff feel relaxed.

I went back onto the ward, and completed Aknesh's honey dressing, I could see how uncomfortable he was as I applied the dressing. Aknesha had brought along his wife Amaul. Amaul was distraught and crying as she sat next to the social worker. Amaul explained that she was struggling as the main carer for Aknesha, and required help explaining she was all on her own. I could tell Amaul found it difficult to make the admission that she struggled to help Aknesha but had finally consented to help.

As I walked out of the bay, I found my patient Lauren standing at the desk, smacking her hands on the counter. Lauren was dressed in two fur coats and a green dressing gown, and her suitcase was filled to the brim.

"I want to go I need to go now! Is anyone listening to me!" I watched as Lauren let out a blood-curdling scream causing all eyes to turn towards her.

"Look, I need to go home," I need to see my children, I need to pick my daughter up!" she yelled.

"Let's go back to your room, there is something I need to tell you," I lied, hoping to distract her from her confused thinking. As I took Lauren to the side room I looked on in shock as I opened her suitcase. So many items fell out of the suitcase. Lauren had packed the suitcase with items she had collected from other patients on the wards, including wallets, jackets, toiletry items.

I called Alina to sit in the side room with Lauren much to her disgust in me taking her away from her cigarettes.

After, I completed the discharge papers for Bill completing my first discharge as a nurse. After I heard a loud shrill scream in the physio room. The physiotherapist team was holding a party, and Arnold had entered the room. When I ran through the double doors, I witnessed Arnold running around with a traffic cone.

"Quick everyone dive under the table there is a bomb," he shouted. I watched as Sister Di ran under the table to emphasize with Arnold, she had a great way of emphasizing with patients.

As I left the physio room, I noticed Lauren standing at the desk with a walking stick in her hand holding it in the air.

"Let me out or I will smash the windows!" she shouted. This was the reality of nursing, and I was only at the beginning.

Chapter 13: Writers' life for me.

After the success of 'The lost Magdalene girl,' I spent six months crafting my next book about my time as a student nurse in London. I spent most evenings and weekends crafting my work and editing all the details. Looking back at my career in working in the hospitals showed how far I had come in the health sector. I started in the hospital as a shy, unworldly, 23-year-old and finished the course confident, and assertive, in responding to critically ill patients and people in emergencies.

I had finally finished my book, and created a glossy front cover depicting a picture of a cartoon nurse on the backdrop of famous London scenery. I had ordered over a hundred paperback copies of my books to use on my promotion journey. I signed up with a publishing initiative called the book fairs. The initiative involved leaving your books in a place such as a forest or shopping centre and for people to find them read it and pass them on. When I signed up for the book fairs, I received a hundred ribbons and stickers and placed them onto my books. I spent a day leaving my books in different areas. I went to my local shopping center and left it on a bench inside, seconds later an elderly man ran after me, "Excuse me sir you've left your book behind!" he shouted. I then left five books on the benches outside a nursing school, I placed three books in a forest. As I arrived home, I looked on in amazement people who discovered my book had posted it on the internet on social media platforms, such as Facebook and Twitter reaching thousands of new readers.

The following week, I was overwhelmed to receive an invitation to a university in London, to discuss my experiences in healthcare, and act as a speaker in a room of five hundred student nurses, on their enrolment and key tutors and professors.

I was so nervous on the day of the talk; I could feel my hands and lips trembling as I walked up the steps to the podium.

I looked out to the sea of nervous faces in the crowd at all the new student nurses who were about to embark on one of the most challenging careers. As I spoke on the microphone, I read the first chapter of a book and I looked on as the student nurses laughed and cheered at my stories. I then completed a question-and-answer session with the students. I was asked what the most challenging moment I had experienced in my time in the hospital. I explained that taking the lead in CPR emergencies was always the most challenging situation, there is so much expectation on your shoulders, and you must focus all your clinical skills on the deteriorating patient. I was then asked what the hardest part was of being a student nurse. I explained that it was working unsociable hours, and not seeing friends or family as often as I wanted to. I explained that the most rewarding part of my career was being with patients at their weakest moments and watching them recover. At the end of the session, I handed out the one hundred paperback versions of my book to the students. I had a great day promoting my book, it was a surreal afternoon giving out my book. I had realized that my dreams were finally coming true.

Chapter 14: Top tips for student nurses

Make sure you revise the basics of human anatomy at the start of the course, you will need this throughout your course, see it as your nursing bible.

Buy a nursing numeracy calculation book to help you through the three numeracy tests you will need over the three years.

Buy a BNF or book about medications as a student nurse you will need to revise and remember the use of over forty medications.

For exams and essays that you need to complete once on placement, draw up a timetable to help you manage a work/life balance.

Build up a good support network with fellow student nurses, you are all going through the same experience and will need support during difficult times.

Ring up your placement setting before you start and ask for a copy of the student handbook, or essential reading for the placement. This shows that you have an interest in your placement area and will help you prepare.

When you start a placement make a note of words you have not come across in the handover sheet and revise their meaning.

Keep a reflection after each shift, write what went well what you would improve next time.

Try to buddy up with other nurses on the ward it can be helpful to see how other nurses work.

Try to get involved in different pathways, attend the theatre for the day, ask to spend a day in the community, it can be helpful to see the full nursing journey.

Try to work and shadow other healthcare professionals such as physiotherapists and occupational therapists it is important to see how other professionals fit into the team.

Try to attend as many ward rounds as possible and walk around the ward with the consultant. Ask questions and be assertive.

Try to attend student briefings that your practice placement manager runs. It is important to connect with other students.

Ask for weekly feedback from your mentor and talk about your strengths and areas that you can work on.

After each shift does something that you enjoy, listen to your favourite music, go for a run or speak to a friend it is important to look after your wellbeing.

If you feel you are not being supported by your mentor or feel bullied in a placement area, you MUST address your concerns. Speak to your ward mentor directly, your placement manager, or your school tutor. This is your nurse training, and you must take control.

Get to grips with the paperwork on the ward and remember to document all tasks.

Be assertive as a student if someone is asking you to complete an activity out of your remit you must say NO.

Make sure you get a good rest during placement; it is important to be refreshed at the start of each shift.

Make sure you eat a balanced diet during your placement, make sure you drink plenty of water. It can be tempted after a stressful shift to reach for sugary food, but it is important to look at alternatives.

Try to complete handovers in as many ways as possible, verbally to your colleagues or over the phone using SBAR this will help with your confidence.

If you feel you are not enjoying your placement, remember your placement time is temporary and you will eventually find other areas you enjoy.

Try to get involved with staff meetings and at the end of the placement be open and honest about any improvements that can be made to support students.

Make a note of all clinical tasks you have completed and record any outstanding that you can bring to future placements.

Try to work with other students on the ward and support them, one day you may be a mentor and it is helpful for your development to support fellow students from the onset.

Ask questions constantly it is the best way you will learn as a student.

Attend as many clinical skills sessions as you can and try to practice the clinical skills at your university center if this is available.

Make use of your library and try to book a tutorial with the librarian about referencing books and writing at level 5/6

If you fail an assignment or did not achieve the grade you wanted ask for feedback or book a tutorial with your tutor to go through areas of improvement.

If you have a placement in the community, make the most of your free time by revising looking up key themes.

Ask to spend a day with a nurse in a specialist field such as a tissue viability nurse or a cardiology nurse it can be a great learning experience.

Try to get involved in CPR opportunities and ward emergencies, stay calm, and follow instructions.

Follow all infection control precautions and encourage visitors to comply with rules.

Try to complete bank shifts as a student it can help to build up your confidence levels and can improve your communication skills.

Try to spend a day with the palliative care team it can be useful to magpie ideas and look at how to respond to difficult conversations.

Ask your mentor if you can have study time each week to help you in your placement.

Try to speak to family members and ward staff over the phone this can be difficult as a student and it is important to practice.

If you fail a placement, see it as a learning experience, not a failure. Look at your targets and plan on completing them.

Make the most of your time off, go to him see a friend it is so important to concentrate on your wellbeing.

Keep up to date with your placement documents.

Make a strict plan when keeping to deadlines plan and write down the steps of how you will achieve the deadline date.

Make friends and family members aware of times when you will be busy and unable to meet.

Be aware of the fire exit on the ward and of any safeguarding policies.

Try to take breaks outside or at least try to get away from the ward/department at breaktimes.

Use nightshifts to ask your mentor to show you outstanding clinical skills and use your nightshift to go through any university paperwork.

If you are not on track to pass your placement, midway ask your mentor to give you clear, measurable, and achievable targets.

Ask if you can shadow the nurse in charge for the day early in your placement this will help you when you take on this role in the future.

Make a list of all important tasks and prioritize the most important tasks.

Always remember as a student you are supernumerary and are not part of the staffing figures.

If a staff member asks you to complete a task but you are not confident say no politely and offer to delegate, the task to someone competent to do so.

If you have people on the ward who are on work experience answer any questions and try to give an overview of your role, it is important to act as a positive role model for others.

Try to attend any in-house training on the ward, it could be learning to use physio equipment or manual handling equipment.

Thank you for reading my book, if you enjoyed it, please leave a review.

For updates follow me on markrog90

The end

www.ingramcontent.com/pod-product-compliance
Lightning Source LLC
Chambersburg PA
CBHW070645220526
45466CB00001B/296